EDITOR'S PREFACE.

THE object of the series of handbooks that is being published under heading of THE ACCOUNTANTS' LIBRARY is to provide, at a reasonable price, detailed information as to the most approved methods of keeping accounts in relation to all the leading classes of industry whose books call for more or less specialised treatment. No such series has hitherto been attempted; but there exist, of course, numerous separate works dealing with the accounts of one particular class of undertaking. These separate works are, however, for the most part either too expensive, or too superficial to answer the purpose that is particularly aimed at by THE ACCOUNTANTS' LIBRARY, which is intended to supply the student with that specialised information which he may require, while at the same time affording to the trader, banker, or manufacturer who is not in a position to secure the fullest information for his purpose, knowledge which can hardly fail to be of the very greatest assistance to him in the correct keeping of his accounts, upon a system specially adapted to his requirements, and therefore involving a minimum expenditure of labour. It is expected that the series will also be found of material assistance to book-keepers of all classes.

Without aiming at giving an exhaustive account of the manner in which each separate business is conducted, the technical points in connection with each industry will receive as much attention as is necessary in order fully to elucidate the system of accounts advocated, while each volume will be the work of one who has made that particular class of accounts more or less a speciality. It is obvious, however, that to enable the necessary ground to be covered in the space available, it is incumbent to assume upon the part of the reader a certain knowledge of general bookkeeping. The extent of the knowledge assumed will vary according to the nature of the class of accounts considered. For example, in the volumes on " Bank Accounts " and " Shipping Accounts " a thorough acquaintance with ordinary double-entry bookkeeping is not unnaturally assumed; but in the case, for instance, of " Auctioneers' Accounts," " Domestic " Tradesmen's Accounts," and other similar volumes, such explanations are included as will enable the ordinarily intelligent reader fully to grasp the methods described even although his knowledge of bookkeeping may be of an elementary description. These explanations are, doubtless, superfluous as far as accountants are concerned, but are necessary to make the volumes of value to the majority of those specially engaged in these particular industries.

To subscribers for the whole series it may be added that, when completed, it will form a most valuable and practically complete library, dealing, at the hands of specialists, with practically every class of accounts, and illustrating the application of the theory of double-entry as described in general works on bookkeeping.

In order to carry out this scheme, arrangements have already been completed for books dealing with the following subjects :—

Agricultural Accounts.
Auctioneers' Accounts.
Australian Mining Accounts.
Bank Accounts.
Bookkeeping and Accounts for Grain, Flour, Hay, Seed, and Allied Trades.
Builders' Accounts.

Building Societies' Accounts.
Co-operative Societies' Accounts.
Cotton Spinners' Accounts.
Drapers' Accounts.
Domestic Tradesmen's Accounts.
Engineers' and Shipbuilders' Accounts.
Gas Accounts.

"THE ACCOUNTANTS' LIBRARY."

VOL. XVIII.

MEDICAL PRACTITIONERS'

ACCOUNTS.

BY

J. HENRY MAY, A.S.A.A

(Joint Author of "Pawnbrokers' Accounts.")

LONDON :

GEE & CO., PRINTERS AND PUBLISHERS, 34 MOORGATE STREET, E.C.

—

1903.

"THE ACCOUNTANTS' LIBRARY."

Edited by the Editor of "The Accountant."

(*To be continued.*)

Hotel Accounts.
Mineral Water Accounts.
Pawnbrokers' Accounts.
Polytechnic Accounts.
Printers' Accounts.
Publishers' Accounts.

Shipping Accounts.
Solicitors' Accounts.
Stockbrokers' Accounts.
Tailors' Accounts.
Theatre Accounts.
Wine Merchants' Accounts.

Arrangements for dealing with other subjects are now in progress, and the Editor wishes to add that he will be glad to receive suggestions and offers from accountants of experience for the undertaking of volumes not yet announced.

34 Moorgate Street,
    London, E.C.
        August 1902.

CONTENTS.

INTRODUCTION.

A CCOUNTING, applied to the Medical Man, does not lend itself to any one universal system. The reason becomes obvious when it is remembered that the clerical work in connection therewith falls, to a very large extent, on the practitioner himself, and in consequence we find the system in each particular case based upon his individual needs, and in some cases on his limited opportunities of entry. As a result, half-a-dozen systems are in use for merely recording Day Book entries; each, in its way, the best under the special circumstances attaching to the practice or the limitations of the practitioner's time.

The want most keenly felt is, no doubt, a system (modified as necessary to each particular practice) for accurately recording bills due, and linking the same to each individual patient in such a fashion as to give all necessary details, and at the same time to ensure accuracy and economy of time and labour. Another object to be kept in view in formulating a system is that of relieving the busy practitioner from a part of the clerical work, at any rate, and allowing of the devolution of such labour to others.

These objects are kept distinctly in view in the suggestions given in the first part of this volume. There will be found sundry methods of Day Book posting in vogue in the profession each of which methods will in turn be found discussed, and the arguments *pro* and *con.* brought forward, leaving the selection of the particular system dependent on the peculiar requirements of the practice.

Given that this prime object (the selection of the most suitable Day Book system) has been accomplished, the Cash Book and Ledger are next discussed. These, of necessity, are designed to combine simplicity with economy of labour, yet enabling the medical man to summarise his total income and expenditure on any balancing date, and therefrom to have regular Profit and Loss Accounts and Balance Sheets prepared.

Full *pro formâ* accounts in illustration of the forms of account books shown are given in each case.

Chapters are subsequently devoted to subjects which accountants find it necessary, at one time or another, to apply themselves—such as "Medical Men's Income Tax," "The Assessment of Practice Values," "Notes on the Collection of Debts Outstanding," &c.

At the end of the volume will be found much general information relating to this honourable profession, which will be found of interest to accountants, and, in some cases (for instance, "Legal Points on a Medical Man's Accounts Owing"), of practical utility.

MEDICAL PRACTITIONERS' ACCOUNTS.

PART I.

CHAPTER I.

THE VISITING LIST.

THE originating source of most of the entries which go to make up the medical man's accounts is the "Visiting List." In it he records his daily visits, as also memoranda relating to the necessity or otherwise for repeating such visits, the despatch of medicines, &c. When properly kept up this book gives him a continuous view of the course of visitation of each patient. It is made up in pocket-book form, and is generally bound up with other important information relating to the Pharmacopæia, &c. It is thus a most valuable pocket companion, and fulfils also the purpose of a recording diary of each case.

The ruling of this book is various. The following ruling is suitable where the list of patients is long : —

Form A.—   VISITING LIST.

Year and Month .... Date																	£	s	d
1st																			
2nd																			
3rd																			
4th																			
5th																			
6th																			
7th																			
8th																			
9th																			
10th																			
11th																			
12th																			

&c., to end of Month

The names of the patients are entered in the diagonal spaces at the top of each leaf, and where (as is often the case) the month's record of visitation can be confined to one opening, the total visits on each round can be clearly seen by running the eye along the line set apart for any particular day. On the other hand, the total visits in any one month made by the practitioner to any one individual case is arrived at by casting up the vertical columns. Where the list of patients is more expanded, a short flyleaf is inserted, ruled as above, but of course without the date column.

A second form of Visiting List is the following :—

Form B.— VISITING LIST.

Year and Month	1	2	3	4	5	6	7	8	9	10	11	12	&c., to end of Month	£ s d
Patient's Name and Address														

It will be observed that in this instance, as in the last, totals for the day (or for a particular patient) can be arrived at without much trouble. No inset, however, is possible with this type of Visiting List, and should the list of patients fill more than one opening, the only alternative is to commence a fresh one.

A third form of Visiting List is the following :—

Form C.— VISITING LIST.

Year and Month	Week ending										Week ending								
Patient's Name and Address	8	9	10	11	12	13	14	£	s	d	15	16	17	18	19	20	21	£ s d

This book is, as a rule, printed on the principle of " one page one week, two weeks to one opening," and is the most popular type of Visiting List in use.

As already stated, the practitioner has to rely very largely upon this valuable diary to keep him in close touch with each individual case, and as to how this is done the following remarks are offered.

To enable the medical man to save both time and economise space in his Visiting List, a system of Signs and Marks has been adopted, in lieu of the ordinary methods of entry. The basis of this system of marks and signs is common to nearly all medical men, there being but modifications of detail in particular cases. This matter, however, we will dismiss by giving one of the published and recognised Lists of Marks, and

EXAMPLE OF VISITING LIST DULY FILLED UP.

Scale	Name and Address	1	2	3	4	5	6	7	8	9	10	11	12	1.
	No.													
A	1 Allen, Mrs., 2 Springfield St.	/	..	..	×	..	..	..	×	..	..	..	×	..
B	2 Briggs, Miss, Snow Hill ..	C./d.	✳	..	..	..	..	..	..	✳	..	..	..	
C	3 Butt, Jno., Victory Rd. ..	/	✳	..	.	..	.	..	..	..	..	/	..	.
A	4 Spencer, Allen, Kelso Rd.	C./d.	..	..	..	..	..	2/4 N.	×	×	×	..	..	..
A	5 Jamieson, Miss, Canada St.	/	×	..	..	×	..	..	..	..	..	/	..	..
A	6 Mathias, Wm., Swan St...	C./d.	..	×	..	..	×	..	..	..	..	✳	..	..
B	7 Allanson, Alf.	..	/	..	..	..	..	C.	..	..	..	..	..	..
C	8 Bateson, Jno., Wilfred Row	..	/	..	..	..	..	..	..	..	✳	..	..	..
A	9 North, Mrs., Hill Villa ..	..	×	×	×	×	×	..	..	×	..	×	×	×
B	10 Younger, Alex., The Mount	..	..	..	..	..	/	×	..	..	×	..	..	..
B	11 Daly, Jno., Circle St. ..	..	..	..	..	..	—	..	..	..	..	..	..	/
C	12 Morden, Mrs., Castle St...	..	..	..	..	..	..	..	C./d.	..	..	✳	..	..
A	13 Jay, Jno., Temple View ..	..	..	..	..	..	..	..	..	/	..	..	..	—
A	14 „ „ Mrs. „ ..	..	..	..	..	..	..	..	..	/	..	..	✳	..
B	15 Jolly, Miss, Temple St. ..	..	..	..	..	..	..	..	..	..	..	..	..	..
A	16 Eben, Mrs., Harthill ..	..	..	..	..	..	..	..	..	..	..	..	..	
A	17 Pick, Mr., Crusoe St. ..	..	..	..	..	..	..	..	..	..	..	..	..	
		3/13/-	4/3/-	10/-	10/	10/-	1/5/6	3/2/6	2/12/-	1/10/6	2/14/-	2/17/-	17/6	18/-

No. 4 item, 7th September : " 2/4," denotes tha

N.B.—The "Scale" column is not usually found in Visiting Lists, an hereinafter shown.

It will be understood that × represents the intersection of the tw append a Visiting List duly filled up as an illustration of the application of the same.

List of "Marks" most commonly used in Visiting List.—

Visit to be made .. .. \	Consultation (at Surgery)	
Visit made .. .. /	"*Concilium domi*" .. C./d.	
Second Visit same day .. X²	Do. (Away) .. .. .. C.	
Third Visit same day .. X³	Night Visit .. .. .. N.	
Visits made, and Medicine to	Special Visit .. .. .. S.	
be sent .. .. .. ✳	Vaccination .. .. .. Vac.	
Do. Medicine sent .. .. ✳	Medicine made up for Caller —	
	Repeat Medicine .. .. R.	

SEPTEMBER 1900.

15	16	17	18	19	20	21	22	23	24	25	26	27	28	29	30	£ s d
..	..	..	..	..	×	..	..	..	..	×	..	..	..	..	..	1 10 0
..	..	✳	..	..	..	..	..	..	..	✳	..	..	..	..	/	4 13 6
..	..	..	..	..	..	R.	..	..	..	..	—	..	..	R.	..	4 8 0
/	..	..	..	..	..	..	..	..	..	..	..	..	..	..	..	2 0 6
..	S.	..	×	..	✳	..	×	..	×	..	×	✳	..	..	×	8 5 0
..	..	/	..	✳	..	..	..	✳	..	..	/	..	..	..	..	3 0 6
..	..	..	..	..	..	..	C./d.	..	..	..	..	/	..	..	..	4 4 0
✳	..	..	..	..	✳	..	..	..	..	✳	..	..	✳	..	..	7 11 0
..	..	..	..	..	..	..	×	..	..	..	×	×	..	..	×	3 5 0
..	..	..	..	..	..	..	..	..	..	..	..	..	..	..	..	1 16 6
..	..	×	..	✳	..	..	✳	..	..	✳	..	..	✳	..	..	4 8 0
✳	..	..	✳	..	..	..	..	✳	..	..	/	×	..	✳	..	10 14 0
..	R.	..	..	..	..	R.	..	..	..	..	..	..	..	R.	..	0 15 0
..	..	✳	..	..	..	..	✳	..	..	..	✳	..	..	✳	..	2 10 0
C./d.	×	..	..	..	×	..	×	..	/	..	..	/	×	..	/	4 14 6
..	..	C.	Vac.	..	..	..	..	..	..	..	..	..	..	..	..	1 3 6
..	..	C./d.	/	..	..	..	..	✳	..	..	..	..	..	✳	..	1 10 6
3/18/-	5/18/-	3/10/-	1/18/6	2/9/-	1/3/-	2/1/-	1/11/-	2/1/-	2/1/6	1/16/-	2/8/6	2/14/6	2/19/6	2/1/-	1/11/-	66 9 6

he visit took place at 2 a.m., and lasted 2 hours.
s given in this case in order to facilitate reference to the Day Book entries

marks \ and /, "Visit to be made" and "Visit made" respectively.

CHAPTER II.

THE DAY BOOKS.

THE Day Books of the medical man are most varied, both in ruling and methods of entry. As no one system can be held to be the best for universal use in the profession, it is now proposed to discuss in turn each of the most useful systems, and to give rulings of the books indispensable to the proper carrying out of the same.

System A.—Utilising the Visiting List as a complete Day Book, and posting direct therefrom to the Ledger.

This is a crude and unsatisfactory method, and is, fortunately, adopted by few practitioners. The following are a few of the objections that should militate against its adoption :—

No Ledger references can be made in the Visiting Lists of the type generally adopted, consequently evidence of items having been posted is usually shown by the rough method of " scoring out."

The Visiting List, not being duplicated in another book, is the only available record, and, in the medical man's absence (with the book), all entries since last posting are unavailable.

The only opportunity of posting the Ledgers is when the medical man is at home, and necessarily this duty will, to a great extent, then fall on himself.

To make the Visiting List a complete posting medium, various entries, beyond its original scope, must be made in it—*e.g.*, Medicines despatched in the practitioner's absence, Consultations at Surgery, &c.

The Visiting List shown on pages 4 and 5 in illustration of the system of marking is written up fully, and shows the total of postings to each patient in the Cash column on the extreme right hand. Whilst written up accurately in this case, its liability to error and the absence of check will quickly become apparent.

In cases, however, where Visiting Lists of the following type are kept, it is possible to post directly from the Visiting List to the Ledger with some show of accuracy. The first three patients' accounts are posted for the sake of illustration.

MEDICAL PRACTITIONERS' ACCOUNTS.

VISITING LIS

Scale	Patient's Name and Address		1	2	3	4	5	6	7	£ s d	Led. Fo.	8	9	10	11	12	13	14	
A	Mrs. Allen	(Address)	/	..	..	X	..	..	..	0 10 0	20	X	..	..	..	X	..	..	
B	Miss Briggs	"	C./d.	✳	..	..	..	..	..	1 16 6	21	..	✳	..	..	..	..	..	
C	John Butt	"	/	✳	..	..	..	..	..	2 7 0	22	..	..	..	/	..	..	—	
A	Allen Spencer	"	C./d.	..	..	..	..	..	2/4 N.	1 0 6	..	..	X	X	X	/	..	..	
A	Miss Jamieson	"	/	X	..	..	X	..	..	0 15 0	..	..	..	..	/	..	..	..	
A	Wm. Mathias	"	C./d.	..	X	..	..	X	..	1 0 6	..	..	..	✳	..	..	✳	
B	Alf. Allanson	"	..	/	..	..	..	..	C.	2 12 6	..	..	..	..	..	..	..	
C	John Bateson	"	..	/	..	..	..	..	..	1 1 0	..	..	..	✳	..	..	..	
A	Mrs. North	"	..	X	X	X	X	X	..	1 5 0	..	..	X	..	X	X	X	..	
B	Alex. Younger	"	..	..	..	..	..	/	X	1 1 0	..	..	..	X	..	..	—	
B	John Daly	"	..	..	..	..	..	—	..	0 5 0	..	..	..	..	..	/	..	
C	Eliz. Morden	"	..	..	..	..	..	..	..	..	C./d.	..	..	✳	..	..	..	..	
A	John Jay	"	..	..	..	..	..	..	..	..	..	/	..	..	—	..		
A	Mrs. Mary Jay	"	..	..	..	..	..	..	..	..	..	..	/	..	✳	..	✳	
B	Miss Jolly	"	..	..	..	..	..	..	..	..	..	..	..	..	..	..	..	C
A	Mrs. Eben	"	..	..	..	..	..	..	..	..	..	..	..	..	..	..	..	
A	Miss Pick	"	..	..	..	..	..	..	..	..	..	..	..	..	..	..	..	
	Month's Total.. £66 9 6									13 14 0									

NOTE.—For convenience of reference a Ledger Folio column has been inserted in eptember 1900.

s d	Led. Fo.	16	17	18	19	20	21	22	£ s d	Led. Fo.	23	24	25	26	27	28	29	30	£ s d	Led. Fo.
10 o	20	..	..	..	..	X	..	..	0 5 0	20	..	..	X	..	..	..	..	..	0 5 0	20
5 6	21	..	✱	..	..	..	..	..	0 15 6	21	..	..	✱	..	..	..	..	/	1 6 0	21
6 o	22	..	..	..	..	..	R.	..	0 5 0	22	..	..	—	..	..	..	R.	..	0 10 0	22
o o	..	..	..	..	..	..	..	..		..	..	..	..	..	..	..	..	..		
5 o	..	S.	..	X	..	✱	..	X	6 2 6	..	..	X	..	X	✱	..	..	X	1 2 6	
15 o	..	..	/	..	✱	..	..	..	0 12 6	..	✱	..	..	/	..	..	..	..	0 12 6	
..	..	..	..	..	..	..	..	C./d.	1 1 0	..	..	..	..	..	/	..	..	..	0 10 6	
12 o	..	..	..	..	✱	..	..	..	1 6 0	..	..	✱	..	..	..	✱	..	..	2 12 0	
o o	..	..	..	..	..	..	X	..	0 5 0	..	..	..	..	X	X	..	..	X	0 15 0	
15 6	..	..	..	..	..	..	..	..		..	..	..	..	..	..	..	..	..		
10 6	..	..	X	..	✱	..	..	✱	2 1 6	..	..	..	✱	..	..	✱	..	..	1 11 0	
14 o	..	..	..	✱	..	..	..	..	1 6 0	..	✱	..	..	/	X	..	✱	..	4 14 0	
7 6	..	R.	..	..	..	..	R.	..	0 5 0	..	..	..	..	..	..	..	R.	..	0 2 6	
o o	..	..	✱	..	..	..	✱	..	0 15 0	..	..	..	..	✱	..	..	✱	..	0 15 0	
1 o	..	X	..	..	..	X	..	X	1 11 6	..	..	/	..	..	/	X	..	/	2 2 0	
..	..	..	C.	Vac	..	..	..	..	1 3 6	..	..	..	..	..	..	..	..	..		
..	..	..	C./d.	/	..	..	..	..	0 15 6	..	✱	..	..	..	..	✱	..	..	0 15 0	
12 o									18 10 6										17 13 0	

iting List shown above.   This column, however, is not usually given in current types.

PATIENTS' LEDGER.

MRS. ALLEN, &c.   Folio 20.

1900			£ s d	£ s d	1900			£ s d
Sept. 1	To Balance owing	√	..	3 1 6	Sept. 5	By Cash ..	C.B.	3 0 0
7	" Bills	V.L.	0 10 0		30	" Balance ..	√	1 11 6
15	" Do.	"	0 10 0					
22	" Do.	"	0 5 0					
30	" Do.	"	0 5 0					
				1 10 0				
			£	4 11 6				£4 11 6
Oct. 1	To Balance due	√	..	1 11 6				

MISS BRIGGS, &c.   Folio 21.

1900			£ s d	£ s d	1900			£ s d
Sept. 7	To Bills ..	V.L.	1 16 6		Sept. 1	By Cash ..	C.B.	1 1 0
15	" Do. ..	"	0 15 6		9	" Do. ..	"	5 0
22	" Do. ..	"	0 15 6		30	" Do. ..	"	3 7 6
30	" Do. ..	"	1 6 0					
				4 13 6				
			£	4 13 6				£4 13 6

JOHN BUTT, &c.   Folio 22.

1900			£ s d	£ s d	1900			£ s d
Sept. 7	To Bills ..	V.L.	2 7 0		Sept. 2	By Cash ..	C.B.	0 5 0
15	" Do. ..	"	1 6 0		30	" Balance ..	√	4 3 0
22	" Do. ..	"	0 5 0					
30	" Do. ..	"	0 10 0					
				4 8 0				
				4 8 0				£4 8 0
Oct. 1	To Balance due	√	..	4 3 0				

When all the accounts in the Ledger have been posted up, the proof of accurate posting will follow the form given under System B (page 18).

System B.—By using the Prescription Book as a Partial Day Book, the rest of the Ledger entries coming from the Visiting List.

The Prescription Book, sometimes called the "Day Book" (a ruling of which will be found in the illustrative accounts following), is a record of the medical and surgical details of each case coming before the medical man. It is not strictly a book of account, though used as such by the majority of practitioners. It is so utilised under System B, becoming the posting medium for Medicines, Consultations, &c., whilst from the Visiting List are posted the daily, weekly, or monthly totals of " visits."

The objections to this system are that there is in this case, as in that of the previous system, no duplication of the Visiting List, and furthermore the absence of a complete single record will be felt. The mere fact of using two books—each, in certain cases, partially—to arrive at the· total postings to the Ledger, will not commend this system to the accountant, owing to the obvious liability to error involved.

As this system is popular amongst medical men, an illustration of its working is now given. The Prescription Day Book, as shown, follows the sequence of entry as given in the details of the illustrative Visiting List (page 4).

For the purpose of following the marks as per Visiting List into their corresponding cash equivalents—as shown in the examples of Day Books hereafter given—the following scale of charges is assumed, not, of course, as being based on either fact or custom : —

	Scale A.	Scale B.	Scale C.
Visit	5/-	10/6	21/-
Medicine and Repeat Mixture	2/6	5/-	5/-
Consultation (at Surgery, &c.)	10/6	21/-	42/-
Do. (away)	21/-	42/-	5/5/-
Special (not fixed)	—	—	
Vac.	2/6	5/-	10/6

While discussing Charges, it is of interest and value to the accountant to know that where the medical man is incapacitated from entering up his books, even from the marked Visiting List, the accountant's clerk is quite available for this purpose, provided such a scale of charges as the above is made out and the Visiting List completed.

Another necessary preliminary to complete the illustration of method of posting under System B is (1) a List of Balances at the commencement of posting; and (2) Items of Cash received from patients during the month. These we suppose to be of the following amounts:—

BALANCES at September 1st.

		£	s	d
No. 1—Scale A—Mrs. Allen		3	1	6
5 A—Miss Jamieson		0	10	6
10 B—Alex. Younger		2	5	0
12 C—Mrs. Morden		8	11	0
16 A—Mrs. Eben		3	5	0
17 A—Mr. Pick		0	10	6
Total ..	£18	3	6

CASH RECEIVED FROM PATIENTS DURING MONTH.

Scale		£	s	d
B—Sept. 1—Miss Briggs (No. 2)		1	1	0
A „ 1—Mr. Spencer („ 4)		0	10	6
A „ 1—W. Mathias („ 6)		0	10	6
C „ 2—Butt („ 3)		0	5	0
A „ 5—Mrs. Allen („ 1)		3	0	0
B „ 9—Briggs („ 2)		0	5	0
C „ 11—Mrs. Morden („ 12)		10	0	0
B „ 13—John Daly („ 11)		0	15	6
A „ 14—Mathias („ 6)		0	2	6
A „ 14—Mrs. Jay („ 14)		0	2	6
B „ 15—Miss Jolly („ 15)		1	11	6
A „ 20—Miss Jamieson („ 5)		7	8	0
A „ 22—Mrs. North („ 9)		2	10	0
A „ 26—Mrs. Jay („ 14)		2	0	0
B „ 30—Miss Briggs („ 2)		3	7	6
Total ..	£33	9	6

Prescription Day Book entries, Sept. 1st to 15ᵗh (inclusive).

PRESCRIPTION DAY BOOK. 205.

				Posting Amount			Ledger Folio	Cash Received		
SEPTEMBER 1st.				£	s	d		£	s	d
Miss Briggs, Snow Hill										
(Details of Case, Formulæ, &c.)	..	..		1	1	0	21	1	1	0
Allen Spencer, Kelso Street										
(Details of Case, &c.)	..	..	..	0	10	6	23	0	10	6
Wm. Mathias, Upper Swan Street										
(Details of Case, &c.)	..	..	..	0	10	6	25	0	10	6
SEPTEMBER 2nd.										
Miss Briggs, Snow Hill										
(Medicine, Formulæ, &c.)	..	..	..	0	5	0	21			
John Butt, Victory Road										
(Medicine, Formulæ, &c.)	..	..	..	0	5	0	22	0	5	0
SEPTEMBER 7th.										
John Daly, Castle Street										
(Medicine, Formulæ, &c.)	..	..	..	0	5	0	30			
SEPTEMBER 8th.										
Mrs. Morden, Castle Street										
(Consultation—Details) ..	..	..	..	2	2	0	31			
SEPTEMBER 9th.										
Miss Briggs, Snow Hill										
(Medicine—Repeat Sept. 2nd) ..	..	..		0	5	0	21	0	5	0
SEPTEMBER 10th.										
Wm. Mathias, Swan Street										
(Medicine, Formulæ, &c.)	..	..	..	0	2	6	25			
J. Bateson, Wilfred Row										
(Medicine, Formulæ, &c.)	..	..	..	0	5	0	27			
SEPTEMBER 11th.										
Mrs. Morden, Castle Street										
(Medicine, Formulæ, &c.)	..	..	..	0	5	0	31	10	0	0
SEPTEMBER 12th.										
Mrs. Jay, Temple View										
(Medicine, Formulæ, &c.)	..	..	..	0	2	6	33			
SEPTEMBER 13th.										
John Jay, Temple View										
(Medicine, Formulæ)	..	..	..	0	2	6	32			
SEPTEMBER 14th.										
John Butt, Victory Road										
(Medicine, Formulæ. &c.)	..	..	..	0	5	0	22			
Wm. Mathias, Swan Street										
(Medicine, Formulæ, &c.)	..	..	..	0	2	6	25	0	2	6
Alex. Younger, The Mount										
(Medicine, Formulæ, &c.)	..	..	..	0	5	0	29			
Mrs. Jay										
(Repeat September 12th)	..	..	..	0	2	6	33	0	2	6
SEPTEMBER 15th.										
John Bateson										
(Repeat September 10th)	..	..	..	0	5	0	27			
Mrs. Morden										
(Repeat September 11th)	..	..	..	0	5	0	31			
Miss Jolly, Temple Street										
(Consultation—Details)	..	..	..	1	1	0	34	1	11	6

NOTE.—The Prescription Book is sometimes used for recording Cash Receipts as well as items chargeable. The Cash Receipts here shown are only such as appertain to the patients whose Day Book postings are given, and are merely memoranda.

PATIENTS' LEDGER.—SYSTEM C.

Method of Posting.—

Visits from Visiting List.   (See page 4.)

Consultations, Medicines, &c., from Prescription Day Book, immediately preceding.

Cash from Cash Book.

MRS. ALLEN, 2 Springfield Street.   Folio 20.

			£ s d					£ s d
Sept. 1	To Balance due ..	✓	3 1 6	Sept. 5	By Cash	C.B.		3 0 0
30	„ Visits	V.L.	1 10 0	„	„ Balance down..	✓		1 11 6
			£4 11 6					£4 11 6
Oct. 1	To Balance due ..	✓	1 11 6					

MISS BRIGGS, Snow Hill.   Folio 21.

			£ s d					£ s d
Sept. 1	To Consultation/d.	P.B.	1 1 0	Sept. 1	By Cash	C.B.		1 1 0
2	„ Medicine ..	„	0 5 0	2	„ Do.	„		0 5 0
9	„ Do. ..	„	0 5 0	30	„ Do.	„		3 7 6
17	„ Do. ..	„	0 5 0					
25	„ Do. ..	„	0 5 0					
30	„ Visits	V.L.	2 12 6					
			£4 13 6					£4 13 6
Oct. 1	To Balance ..							

JOHN BUTT, Victory Road.   Folio 22.

			£ s d					£ s d
Sept. 2	To Medicine ..	P.B.	0 5 0	Sept. 2	By Cash	C.B.		0 5 0
14	„ Do. ..	„	0 5 0	30	„ Balance due ..	✓		4 3 0
21	„ Do. ..	„	0 5 0					
26	„ Do. ..	„	0 5 0					
29	„ Do. ..	„	0 5 0					
30	„ Visits	V.L.	3 3 0					
			£4 8 0					£4 8 0
Oct. 1	To Balance due ..	✓	4 3 0					

ALLEN SPENCER, 13 Kelso Street.   Folio 23.

			£ s d				£ s d
Sept. 1	To Con./d.	P.B.	0 10 6	Sept. 1	By Cash	C.B.	0 10 6
30	„ Visits	V.L.	1 0 0	30	„ Balance due	✓	1 10 0
	„ Special Visit	„	0 10 0				
			£2 0 6				£2 0 6
Oct. 1	To Balance due	✓	1 10 0				

MISS JAMIESON, 3 Canada Street.   Folio 24.

			£ s d				£ s d
Sept. 1	To Balance	✓	0 10 6	Sept. 30	By Cash	C.B.	7 8 0
16	„ Special Operation	P.B.	5 5 0	„	„ Balance due	✓	1 7 6
20	„ Medicine	„	0 2 6				
27	„ Do.	„	0 2 6				
30	„ Visits	„	2 15 0				
			£8 15 6				£8 15 6
Oct. 1	To Balance due	✓	1 7 6				

WILLIAM MATHIAS, Swan Street.   Folio 25.

			£ s d				£ s d
Sept. 1	To Con./d.	P.B.	0 10 6	Sept. 1	By Cash	C.R.	0 10 6
10	„ Medicine	„	0 2 6	14	„ Do.	„	0 2 6
14	„ Do.	„	0 2 6	30	„ Balance due	✓	2 7 6
19	„ Do.	„	0 2 6				
23	„ Do.	„	0 2 6				
30	„ Visits	V.L.	2 0 0				
			£3 0 6				£3 0 6
Oct. 1	To Balance	✓	2 7 6				

ALFRED ALLANSON, Upper Swan Street.   Folio 26.

			£ s d				
Sept. 22	To Con./d.	P.B.	1 1 0				
30	„ Visits	V.B.	1 1 0				
	„ Do. (Special)	„	2 2 0				
			£4 4 0				

JOHN BATESON, Wilfred Row.   Folio 27.

				£	s	d			
Sept. 10	To Medicine	..	P.B.	0	5	0			
15	„ Do. ..	..	„	0	5	0			
19	„ Do. ..	..	„	0	5	0			
24	„ Do. ..	..	„	0	5	0			
28	„ Do. ..	..	„	0	5	0			
30	„ Visits ..	..	V.L.	6	6	0			
				£7	11	0			

MRS. NORTH, Hill Villa.   Folio 28.

				£	s	d					£	s	d
Sept. 30	To Visits ..	..	V.L.	3	5	0	Sept. 22	By Cash ..	..	C.B.	2	10	0
							30	„ Balance	..	✓	0	15	0
				£3	5	0					£3	5	0
Oct. 1	To Balance	..	✓	0	15	0							

ALEXANDER YOUNGER, The Mount.   Folio 29.

				£	s	d			
Sept. 1	To Balance due ..	✓		2	5	0			
14	„ Medicine	..	P.B.	0	5	0			
30	„ Visits ..	..	V.L.	1	11	6			
				£4	1	6			

JOHN DALY, Circle Street.   Folio 30.

				£	s	d					£	s	d
Sept. 6	To Medicine	..	P.B.	0	5	0	Sept. 13	By Cash ..	..	C.B.	0	15	6
19	„ Do.	..	„	0	5	0	30	„ Balance	..	✓	3	12	6
22	„ Do.	..	„	0	5	0							
25	„ Do.	..	„	0	5	0							
28	„ Do.	..	„	0	5	0							
30	„ Visits ..	..	V.B.	3	3	0							
				£4	8	0					£4	8	0
Oct. 1	To Balance due ..	✓		3	12	6							

ELIZABETH MORDEN (Mrs.), Castle Street.   Folio 31.

				£	s	d						£	s	d
Sept. 1	To Balance due ..		√	8	11	0	Sept. 10	By Cash ..	..	C.B.		10	0	0
8	„ Con./d.	..	P.B.	2	2	0		„ Balance	..	√		9	5	0
11	„ Medicine	..	„	0	5	0								
15	„ Do.	..	„	0	5	0								
18	„ Do.	..	„	0	5	0								
23	„ Do.	..	„	0	5	0								
29	„ Do.	..	„	0	5	0								
30	„ Visits ..	..	V.L.	7	7	0								
				£19	5	0						£19	5	0
Oct. 1	To Balance	..	√	9	5	0								

JOHN JAY, Temple View.   Folio 32.

				£	s	d					
Sept. 13	To Medicine	..	P.B.	0	2	6					
16	„ Do.	..	„	0	2	6					
21	„ Do.	..	„	0	2	6					
29	„ Do.	..	„	0	2	6					
30	„ Visits ..	..	V.B.	0	5	0					
				£0	15	0					

Mrs. MARY JAY, Temple View.   Folio 33.

				£	s	d						£	s	d
Sept. 12	To Medicine	..	P.B.	0	2	6	Sept. 14	By Cash ..	..	C.B.		0	2	6
14	„ Do.	..	„	0	2	6	26	„ Do. ..	..	„		2	0	0
17	„ Do.	..	„	0	2	6	30	„ Balance	..	√		0	7	6
21	„ Do.	..	„	0	2	6								
26	„ Do.	..	„	0	2	6								
29	„ Do.	..	„	0	2	6								
30	„ Visits ..	..	V.L.	1	15	0								
				£2	10	0						£2	10	0
Oct. 1	To Balance	..	√	0	7	6								

Miss JOLLY, Temple Street.   Folio 34.

				£	s	d						£	s	d
Sept. 15	To Con./d.	..	P.B.	1	1	0	Sept. 15	By Cash ..	..	C.B.		1	11	6
30	„ Visits ..	..	V.L.	3	13	6	30	„ Balance	..	√		3	3	0
				£4	14	6						£4	14	6
Oct. 1	By Balance	..	√	3	3	0								

MRS. EBEN, Hart Hill.   Folio 35.

				£	s	d				
Sept.	1	To Balance	..	✓	3	5	0			
	17	„ Con. ..	..	P.B.	1	1	0			
	18	„ Vac. ..	..	„	0	2	6			
	30	„ Visits ..	..	V.L.						
				£4	8	6				

MR. MATTHEW PICK, Crusoe Street.   Folio 36.

				£	s	d			
Sept.	1	To Balance	..	0	10	6			
	17	„ Con. ..	.. P B.	0	10	6			
	23	„ Medicine	.. „	0	2	6			
	28	„ Do.	.. „	0	2	6			
	30	„ Visits ..	.. V.L.	0	15	0			
				£2	1	0			

SUMMARY OF MONTH'S ENTRIES.					BALANCES AT OCTOBER 1st.						
		£	s	d	Folio					£	s	d
Balances at September 1st	..	18	3	6	20	Allen ..	..	..	..	1	11	6
Total of Visiting List	..	66	9	6	21	Briggs ..	..	..	..	—		
					22	Butt ..	..	..	..	4	3	0
		84	13	0	23	Spencer	..	..	..	1	10	0
Cash received during Month	..	33	9	6	24	Jamieson	..	..	..	1	7	6
					25	Mathias..	..	..	..	2	7	6
					26	Allanson	..	..	..	4	4	0
					27	Bateson..	..	..	..	7	11	0
					28	North ..	..	..	..	0	15	0
					29	Younger	..	..	..	4	1	6
					30	Daly ..	..	..	..	3	12	6
					31	Morden..	..	..	..	9	5	0
					32	Jay ..	..	..	..	0	15	0
					33	„	..	..	..	0	7	6
					34	Jolly ..	..	..	..	3	3	0
					35	Eben	..	..	..	4	8	6
					36	Pick ..	..	..	..	2	1	0
Balances as per above Accounts	£51	3	6						£51	3	6

An alternative ruling for a Patients' Ledger will be found under the head of "Filing Systems," page 36.

Under this system it is understood that although the Prescription Day Book is used as a posting medium for consultations and medicines only, it is also utilised by the practitioner as a memorandum book containing particulars relating to the medical aspect of his cases for record and future reference, as also of cash details. All such items of memoranda are not, of course, posted, a tick being usually made in the folio column provided, in lieu of the usual posting reference.

System C.—All chargeable items being entered up in a separate Day Book, and the same summarised and posted monthly.

This method is distinctly time-saving, and yet allows of accuracy and sufficient detail being shown to stamp it as being one of the best of current systems.

The procedure in carrying it out is as follows :—

Visiting List.—

This is entered up as usual, and the chargeable entries are duplicated into a conveniently ruled book called the " Summary Book."

Prescription Day Book.—

This book is entered up as usual, and fulfils its legitimate object in the medical man's scheme of accounts—viz., the recording of private and professional information regarding his patients, the formulæ of prescriptions, details of consultations, &c. Chargeable items are, however, duplicated regularly into the Summary Book, which is so arranged that it can be written up to show the regular and continuous course of the practitioner's bills as they accrue.

The advantages of this system are obvious :—

(a) The Visiting List is duplicated, and that without much extra trouble, so that in the medical man's absence his outstanding accounts, written up to date, can be seen.

(*b*) A little work each day avoids the periodical accumulations of clerical work which generally fall to the medical man's lot.

(*c*) All chargeable items being separated from the *private* details of the Prescription Book, and placed in a separate book of *account* (and this only), the medical man can, without the least compunction, depute any trustworthy third party to write up his books, whether in his absence or otherwise.

SUMMARY BOO[K]

Scale	No.	Patient's Name and Address	1	2	3	4	5	6	7	8	9	10	11	12	13
A	1	Mrs. Allen ..	5/-	..	..	5/-	..	..	..	5/-	..	..	..	5/-	..
B	2	Miss Briggs ..	21/-	15/6	..	..	..	..	..	..	15/6	..	..	..	..
C	3	John Butt	21/-	26/-	..	..	..	..	..	..	..	..	21/-	..	..
A	4	Spencer, A. ..	10/6	..	..	..	..	..	10/-	5/-	5/-	5/-	..	..	..
A	5	Miss Jamieson ..	5/-	5/-	..	..	5/-	..	..	..	..	5/-	..	..	..
A	6	Wm. Mathias ..	10/6	..	5/-	..	..	5/-	..	..	7/6	..	..	..	..
B	7	A. Allanson ..	..	10/6	..	..	..	..	42/-	..	..	..	..	..	..
C	8	J. Bateson ..	..	21/-	..	..	..	..	..	..	..	26/-	..	..	..
A	9	Mrs. North ..	..	5/-	5/-	5/-	5/-	5/-	..	..	5/-	..	5/-	5/-	5/-
B	10	A. Younger ..	..	..	..	..	..	10/6	10/6	..	..	10,6	..	5/-	5/-
B	11	J. Daly ..	..	..	..	..	..	5/-	..	..	..	..	..	..	10/6
C	12	Mrs. Morden ..	..	..	..	..	..	..	..	42/-	..	..	26/-	..	10/6
A	13	J. Jay ..	..	..	..	..	..	..	..	..	..	..	..	..	2/6
A	14	Mrs. Jay ..	..	..	..	..	..	..	..	..	5/-	..	..	7/6	..
B	15	Miss Jolly ..	..	..	..	..	..	..	..	..	..	5/-	..	7/6	..
A	16	Mrs. Eben ..	..	..	..	..	..	..	..	..	..	..	..	..	..
A	17	Mr. Pick ..	..	..	..	..	..	..	..	..	..	..	..	..	..
			3/13/-	4/3/-	10/-	10/-	10/-	1/5/6	3/2/6	2/12/-	1/10/6	2/14/-	2/17/-	17/6	18/-

It will be observed that by this system a great saving of Ledger space is effected, and a summary of each month's totals easily arrived at. Moreover, each opening (usually containing space for one month) is capable of easy proof, as by casting up the daily totals, and adding these together, an agreement should be found with the total of the individual patients' monthly bills.

A still more extended and detailed method of carrying out this system is to show on separate lines, as and where neces-

(*d*) All the entries making up his chargeable items being in one book, a summarising of the business may be effectually and easily dealt with.

In illustration of the system, it is now proposed to give *pro formâ* accounts, based, as in the previous example, on the Visiting List (duly written up) given on page 4.

The shortest form of Summary Book entry is the following :—

DICINES, &c.

16	17	18	19	20	21	22	23	24	25	26	27	28	29	30	£ s d	Led.Fo.
..	..	..	..	5 -	..	..	..	..	5/-	..	..	..	..	..	1 10 0	A
..	15/6	..	..	..	..	..	..	..	15 6	..	..	..	..	10/6	4 13 6	B
..	..	..	..	..	5/-	..	..	..	..	5/-	..	..	5/-	..	4 8 0	B
5/5/-	..	..	..	7/6	..	5/-	..	5/-	..	5/-	7/6	..	..	5/-	2 0 6	S
..	..	5/-	7/6	..	..	..	7/6	..	..	..	10/6	..	..	..	8 5 0	J
..	..	26/-	..	..	..	..	..	26/-	..	..	..	..	26/-	..	3 0 6	M
..	..	..	26/-	..	..	..	..	..	..	..	..	26/-	..	..	4 4 0	A
..	26/-	..	..	..	5/-	..	..	..	..	5/-	..	..	..	..	7 11 0	B
..	..	..	..	..	..	15/6	..	..	15/6	..	5/-	..	5/-	..	3 5 0	N
..	..	..	..	..	26/-	..	..	..	..	..	21/-	..	..	..	1 16 6	Y
..	21/-	..	..	..	..	..	..	..	..	5/-	..	15/6	..	..	4 8 0	D
2/6	..	..	..	..	5/-	..	26/-	..	..	..	..	..	..	..	10 14 0	M
..	7/6	..	..	..	..	..	..	..	..	7/6	..	..	5/-	..	0 15 0	J
10/6	..	2/6	..	..	..	..	..	10/6	..	..	..	..	..	..	2 10 0	I
..	..	..	15/6	10/6	..	10/6	..	..	..	..	10/6	10/6	..	10/6	4 14 6	L
..	..	..	..	..	..	..	7/6	..	..	..	..	..	..	5/-	1 3 6	E
..	..	5/-	..	..	..	..	..	..	..	..	..	7/6	..	..	1 10 6	P
5/18/-	3/10/-	1/18/6	2/9/-	1/3/-	2/1/-	1/11/-	2/1/-	2/1/6	1/16/-	2/8/6	2/14/6	2/19/6	2/1/-	1/11/-	£66 9 6	

sary, the amounts charged under specific heads, to illustrate which the following account is given.

Whilst illustrating this extended method of entering, opportunity is taken to illustrate a manner of entering up which is observed by some practitioners—viz., deducting from the monthly amount chargeable to each patient items of cash received during the month on account of fees, and posting the *net* amount remaining to the Ledger.

#	Patient's Name and Address		1	2	3	4	5	6	7	8	9	10	11	12	13	14	15	16
1	Mrs. Allen, 2 Springfield St.	Visits	5/-	..	..	5/-	..	..	..	5/-	..	..	..	5/-	..	..	..	..
2	Miss Briggs, Snow Hill ..	Con.	21/-	..	..	..	..	..	..	..	..	..	..	..	..	..	..	..
		Visits	..	10/6	..	..	..	..	..	..	..	10/6	..	..	..	..	..	..
		Med	..	5/-	..	..	..	..	..	..	..	5/-	..	..	..	..	..	..
3	Mr. John Butt, Victory Rd.	Visits	21/-	21/-	..	..	..	..	..	..	..	..	21/-	..	..	..	..	..
		Med.	..	5/-	..	..	..	..	..	..	..	..	..	..	..	5/-	..	..
4	Mr. A. Spencer, Kelso Rd.	Con./d.	10/6	..	..	..	..	..	..	..	..	..	..	..	..	..	..	..
		NightV.	..	..	..	..	..	..	10/-	..	..	..	..	..	..	..	..	..
		Visits	..	..	..	..	..	..	..	5/-	5/-	5/-	..	..	..	..	5/-	..
5	Miss Jamieson, Canada St.	Visits	5/-	5/-	..	..	5/-	..	..	..	..	..	5/-	..	..	..	..	5/5
		Special	..	..	..	..	..	..	..	..	..	..	..	..	..	..	..	..
6	Wm. Mathias, Swan St. ..	Con./d.	10/6	..	..	..	..	..	..	..	..	..	..	..	..	..	..	..
		Visits	..	..	5/-	..	..	5/-	..	..	..	5/-	..	..	..	5/-	..	..
		Med.	..	..	..	..	..	..	..	..	..	2/6	..	..	..	2/6	..	..
7	Alf. Allanson, Swan St. ..	Visit	..	10/6	..	..	..	..	..	..	..	..	..	..	..	..	..	..
		Con.	..	..	..	..	..	42/-	..	..	..	..	..	..	..	..	..	..
		Con./d.	..	..	..	..	..	..	..	..	..	..	..	..	..	..	..	..
8	John Bateson, Wilfred Rd.	Visit	..	21/-	..	..	..	..	..	..	..	21/.	..	..	..	21/-	..	..
		Med.	..	..	..	..	..	..	..	..	..	5/-	..	..	..	5/-	..	..
9	Mrs. North, Hill Villa ..	Visits	..	5/-	5/-	5/-	5/-	5/-	..	..	5/-	..	5/-	5/-	5/-	..	..	..
10	Mr. A. Younger, The Mount	Visits	..	..	..	..	..	10/6	10/6	..	..	10/6	..	..	..	..	..	..
		Med.	..	..	..	..	..	..	..	..	..	..	..	..	5/-	..	..	..
11	John Daly, Circle Street..	Med.	..	..	..	..	..	5/-	..	..	..	..	..	..	..	..	..	..
		Visit	..	..	..	..	..	..	..	..	..	..	..	..	10/6	..	..	..
12	Mrs. Morden, Castle St. ..	Con./d.	..	..	..	..	..	..	..	42/-	..	..	..	..	..	..	..	..
		Visit	..	..	..	..	..	..	..	..	..	..	21/-	..	..	..	21/-	..
		Med.	..	..	..	..	..	..	..	..	..	..	5/-	..	..	..	5/-	..
13	John Jay, Temple View ..	Visits	..	..	..	..	..	..	..	..	5/-	..	..	..	..	..	..	..
		Med.	..	..	..	..	..	..	..	..	..	..	..	..	2/6	..	..	2/6
14	Mrs. Jay, Do. ..	Visit	..	..	..	..	..	..	..	..	5/-,	..	5/-	..	5/-	..	..	..
		Med.	..	..	..	..	..	..	..	..	..	..	2/6	..	2/6	..	..	..
15	Miss Jolly, Temple Street	Con./d	..	..	..	..	..	..	..	..	..	..	..	..	..	..	21/-	..
		Visits	..	..	..	..	..	..	..	..	..	..	..	..	..	..	..	10/6
16	Mrs. Eben, Hart Hill ..	Con.	..	..	..	..	..	..	..	..	..	..	..	..	..	..	..	..
		Vac.	..	..	..	..	..	..	..	..	..	..	..	..	..	..	..	..
17	Mr. Pick, Crusoe Street ..	Con./d.	..	..	..	..	..	..	..	..	..	..	..	..	..	..	..	..
		Visit	..	..	..	..	..	..	..	..	..	..	..	..	..	..	..	..

N.B.—Where, in cases such as that of Mrs. Allen, given above, the Cash received
both items in lieu of the n

SEPTEMBER 1900. Page 27.

MEDICINES, &c.

19	20	21	22	23	24	25	26	27	28	29	30	31	Items of Fees	Month's Fees	Discount, &c.	Dates Cash Rec'ved	Month's Cash	Balance Posted	Letter in Ledg.
													£ s d	£ s d			£ s d	£ s d	
													1 10 0			5th	3 0 0	Bills 1 10 0	
..	5/-	..	..	..	..	5/-	..	..	..	..	..	..		1 10 0	..			Cash 3 0 0	A
..	..	..	..	..	..		..	..	..	..	..		1 1 0	2 12 6		1st	1 1 0		
..	..	..	..	..	..	10/6	..	..	..	..	10/6	..	2 12 6		..	9th	0 5 0		
..	..	..	..	..	..	5/-	..	..	..	..	..	..	1 0 0	4 13 6	..	30th	3 7 6	..	B
																	4 13 6		
..	..	5/-	..	..	..	..	5/-	..	..	5/-	..	..	3 3 0		..	2nd	0 5 0		
													1 5 0	4 8 0	..		..	4 3 0	B
..	..	..	..	..	..	..	..	..	..	..	..	..	0 10 6		..	1st	0 10 6		
..	..	..	..	..	..	..	..	..	..	..	..	..	0 10 0						
..	..	..	..	..	..	..	..	..	..	..	..	..	1 0 0	2 0 6	..		..	1 10 0	S
..	5/-	..	5/-	..	5/-	..	5/-	5/-	..	..	5/-	..	2 15 0		..	20th	7 8 0		
..	2/6	..	..	..	..	..	..	2/6	..	..	..	..	5 5 0						
													0 5 0	8 5 0	..		..	0 17 0	J
5/-	..	..	5/-	..	5/-	..	..	..	..	..	..	..	0 10 6		..	1st	0 10 6		
2/6	..	..	2/6	..	..	..	..	..	..	..	..	..	2 0 0		..	14th	0 2 6		
..	..	..	..	..	..	..	..	..	..	..	..	..	0 10 0	3 0 6	..		0 13 0	2 7 6	M
..	..	..	..	..	..	..	10/6	..	..	..	..	..	1 1 0						
..	..	..	..	..	..	..	..	..	..	..	..	..	2 2 0						
..	..	21/-	..	..	..	..	..	..	..	..	..	..	1 1 0	4 4 0	..		..	4 4 0	A
21/-	..	..	..	..	21/-	..	..	..	21/-	..	..	..	6 6 0						
5/-	..	..	..	..	5/-	..	..	..	5/-	..	..	..	1 5 0	7 11 0	..		..	7 11 0	B
..	..	5/-	..	..	..	..	5/-	5/-	..	..	5/-	..	3 5 0		..	22nd	2 10 0	0 15 0	N
													1 11 6	3 5 0					
..	..	..	..	..	..	..	..	..	..	..	..	..	0 5 0	1 16 6	..		..	1 16 6	Y
5/-	..	..	5/-	..	..	5/-	..	..	5/-	..	..	..	1 5 0		..	13th	0 15 6		
10/6	..	..	10/6	..	..	10/6	..	..	10/6	..	..	..	3 3 0	4 8 0			..	3 12 6	D
..	..	..	..	21/-	..	..	21/-	21/-	..	21/-	..	..	2 2 0		..	10th	10 0 0		
..	..	..	..	5/-	..	..	..	..	..	5/-	..	..	7 7 0						
													1 5 0	10 14 0	..		..	0 14 0	M
..	..	2/6	..	..	..	..	..	..	2/6	..	..	..	0 5 0						
													0 10 0	0 15 0	..		..	0 15 0	J
..	..	5/-	..	..	..	5/-	..	..	5/-	..	..	..	1 15 0		..	14th	0 2 6		
..	..	2/6	..	..	..	2/6	..	..	2/6	..	..	..	0 15 0	2 10 0	..	26th	2 0 0	0 7 6	J
..	10/6	..	10/6	..	10/6	..	10/6	10/6	..	10/6	..		1 1 0		..	15th	1 11 6		
													3 13 6	4 14 6			..	3 3 0	J
/6	..	..	..	..	..	..	..	..	..	..	..	..	1 1 0						
													0 2 6	1 3 6	..		..	1 3 6	E
/-	..	..	5/-	..	..	..	..	5/-	..	..	..	..	0 10 6						
..	..	..	2/6	..	..	..	..	2/6	..	..	..	..	0 15 0						
													0 5 0	1 10 6	..		..	1 10 6	P
														66 9 6					

Account is of larger amount than the Month's Charges, it is no difficult matter to post amount, as in other cases.

It is found in practice that the Summary Book is more valuable when each page is ruled into sections, as in the illustration. This should allow of, say, three lines for the details of each patient's bill—*i.e.,* for " Visits," " Medicines," and " Consultations." If one page of each opening in the Summary Book is reserved for patients of this class, the other page can be utilised for recording the " one visit " patients where but one line would be required for each name. -

The Visiting List is duly written up, either regularly or at the month end, into the Summary Book, and all daily charges —such as Medicines, Consultations, &c.—can be debited straightway to each patient as the same accrue.

The type of Ledger most suitable for medical men who adopt the system of posting monthly amounts to each patient is the " index " pattern. An example of this is now given, showing the postings from the month's Summary of Charges preceding : —

PATIENTS' LEDGER—INDEX PATTERN—FOR MONTHLY POSTING.

Patient's Name and Address	Accounts Outstanding at Jan. 1	Jan.	Feb.	Mar.	April	May	June	Accounts Rendered July 1	Cash Received	Accounts Outstanding at July 1	July	Aug.	Sept.	Oct.	Nov.	Dec.	Accounts Rendered Jan. 1	Cash Received	Accounts Outstanding at Jan. 1
	£ s d	£ s d	£ s d	£ s d	£ s d	£ s d	£ s d	£ s d	£ s d	£ s d	£ s d	£ s d	£ s d	£ s d	£ s d	£ s d	£ s d	£ s d	£ s d
Allen, Mrs. &c.													1 10 0						
Allanson, Alf. "													4 4 0						
Briggs, Miss "													4 13 6						
Butt, John "													4 8 0						
Bateson, Jno. "													7 11 0						
Daly, John "													4 8 6						
Eben, Mrs. "													1 3 6						
Jamieson, Miss "													8 5 0						
Jay, Jno. "													0 15 0						
" Mrs.													2 10 0						
Jolly, Miss "													4 14 6						
Morden, Mrs. "													10 14 0						
Mathias, Mr. "													3 0 6						
North, Mrs. "													3 5 0						
Pick, Mr. "													1 10 6						
Spencer, Allen "													2 0 6						
Younger, Alex. "													1 16 6						

NOTE.—This Ledger is, of course, arranged that all accounts under each alphabetical letter are set apart in special sections, and not as shown above.

The Ledger could also be arranged for *weekly* posting, the Visiting List (Style C) being the originating Day Book.

On the basis of a known number of patients, the above book can be made to order to last a specified period, the names of the months being printed in as required.

In cases where medical men receive part of their fees by *instalments* (as in some working-class practices), a "Cash Summary Book," after the style of that given on page 20, is useful, and enables the practitioner to easily arrive at periodical totals of cash received from patients.

The ordinary form of Index Ledger is not shown, being merely an ordinary Ledger with index enabling all accounts of one initial letter to be placed on one page or in one section.

System D.—All chargeable items, in proper sequence and priority, being entered separately in a Day Book, and posted separately into the Ledger.

This is the longest, and possibly the most methodical, plan for posting; but because of the time occupied in its proper carrying out, is only used by a minority of practitioners. The procedure under this system is as follows:—

(a) *One* Day Book is used.

(b) Visits when made are entered in this book, and the posting amount filled in.

(c) Medicines or prescriptions also are entered as given or despatched, with the amount chargeable.

(d) Consultations, operations, &c., are also entered under their proper date, with corresponding posting amount.

It will thus be seen that this book contains a jumble of all the practitioner's records, and it would be a somewhat difficult matter to get out summarised totals at any particular date. Indeed, in cases where this system is in vogue, it is not at all an uncommon occurrence for the book to be posted up to the Ledger only at such times as any particular account is required to be rendered. In other cases the medical man does not post any details to the Ledger, but by a system of linking all the items appertaining to each patient (after the fashion of the commercial Press Copy Book) he, as occasion requires, gets out the total up to a certain date, and enters it in his Ledger in one amount, only particularising it by a note of the date up to which it is inclusive.

Where it is required to have books designed to show separately every visit, consultation, and, indeed, every chargeable item coming in the medical man's practice, the following rulings are suggested as being of a useful and popular type:—

A.—Prescription Book.—

This is not a book of account, and consequently does not concern accountants intimately. Nevertheless, a few remarks upon it will possibly be advantageous. Most books of this type in use are merely plain Journals, the divisions between each prescription being roughly made by hand, and in some cases, on the medicines being paid for at the time, are scored through as evidence of the fact. The following ruling will be of undoubted advantage in most cases : —

PRESCRIPTION BOOK.

(To contain details of all other chargeable items and notes on cases.)

(Day and Date). Page 45.

Name and Address of Patient	Remarks on Case, Formulæ of Prescription, Details of Visit, &c., &c.	Amount Charged	Cash at time	Amount to Ledger	Ledger Folio
		£ s d	£ s d	£ s d	

PRESCRIPTION BOOK (for Professional details only).

(Day and Date). Page 45.

Name and Address of Patient	Professional Details of Consultations and Medicines, &c., &c.	To Medicine Book Folio	To Visits Book Folio

When this type of Prescription Book is used, it is necessary to have another Day Book, to which chargeable items from the Prescription Book are posted in as terse a form as possible, from which they are taken to the Ledger. An obvious advantage of this method is that nothing but accounting matter is shown in the books of account. The further advantage is also secured of enabling the posting items of the Day Book to be so freed from detail *that the plan of " one line, one entry "* can well be observed.

PRESCRIPTION BOOK.—A book specially adapted for recording the formulæ of prescriptions, and, for this purpose alone, is sold by account book makers. Its size is usually that which allows of each page being 16" by 13". The ruling is merely that of lines intersecting and dividing the pages into squares, each square space being intended to hold the record of one prescription.

Where a separate Medicine Day Book is kept, the following ruling will be found suitable :—

MEDICINE DAY BOOK.

Date	Folio in Prescription Book	To whom despatched	Address	Remarks	£ s d	Ledger Folio

In the " Remarks " column will be noted any memoranda as to whether paid for or not, as to special mode of delivery, &c. An alternative method of showing cash receipts for medicine is to have a column ruled specially for the purpose.

Another ruling of a book for recording the posting items for Consultations, Visits, and Medicines is the following. (This book can be written up from the Prescription Book, &c., on the " one line, one entry " system.) :—

(Day and Date).

Prescrip-tion Book Folio or No.	Cash Received	Details	Visits, Consulta-tions, &c.	Medicines	Amount to Ledger	Folio
	£ s d		£ s d	£ s d	£ s d	

PRESCRIPTION DAY BOOK (used as posting medium to Ledger).
Written up as per Visiting List, page 4.

SEPTEMBER 1st.

Name and Address of Patient	Professional Details	Cash Received	Charges		To Ledger	Folio
			Med.	Con., Vis., &c.		
		£ s d	£ s d	£ s d	£ s d	
Allen, Mrs. (Address)	Visit, &c. .. (Details)	..	..	0 5 0	0 5 0	72
Briggs, Miss ,,	Con /d. .. (Details)	1 1 0	..	1 1 0	..	81
Butt, John ,,	Visit (Details)	..	..	1 1 0	1 1 0	82
Spencer, A. ,,	Con./d. .	0 10 6	..	0 10 6	..	83
Jamieson, Miss ,,	Visit .. (Details)	..	..	0 5 0	0 5 0	84
Mathias, W. ,,	Con. .. (Details)	0 10 6	..	0 10 6	..	86

SEPTEMBER 2nd.

Name and Address of Patient	Professional Details	Cash Received	Med.	Con., Vis., &c.	To Ledger	Folio
Briggs, Miss (Address)	Visit&Medicine (Details)	..	0 5 0	0 10 6	0 15 6	90
Butt, John ,,	Visit&Medicine (Details)	0 5 0	0 5 0	1 1 0	1 1 0	91
Jamieson, Miss ,,	Visit .. (Details)	.	..	0 5 0	0 5 0	98
Allanson, A. ,,	Visit .. (Details)	..	..	0 10 6	0 10 6	99
Bateson, J. ,,	Visit .. (Details)	..	..	1 1 0	1 1 0	100
North, Mrs. ,,	Visit .. (Details)	..	..	0 5 0	0 5 0	101
		£2 7 0	£0 10 0	£7 6 0	£7 16 0	

PRESCRIPTION BOOK (not used as Ledger posting medium).

Written up as per Visiting List, page 4.   (Professional Details only).

SEPTEMBER 1st.   Page 55.

Name and Address of Patient	Professional Details	Day Book
Mrs. Allen, 2 Springfield Street	Visit, &c.	49
Miss Briggs, Snow Hill	Consultation/d. (Particulars)	"
John Butt, Victory Road	Visit (Details)	"
Allen Spencer, Kelso Street	Consultation/d. (Particulars)	"
Miss Jamieson, Canada Street	Visit (Details)	"
Wm. Mathias, Swan Street	Consultation (Details)	"

SEPTEMBER 2nd.

Name and Address of Patient	Professional Details	Day Book
Miss Briggs, Snow Hill	Visit and Medicine (Details and Formulæ, &c.)	50
John Butt, Victory Road	Visit and Medicine (Particulars and Formulæ)	"
Miss Jamieson, Canada Street	Visit (Details)	"
Allanson, Alf. Swan Street	Do. do.	"
John Bateson, Wilfred Row	Do. do.	"
Mrs. North, Hill Villa	Do. do.	"

DAY BOOK.

SEPTEMBER 1st.   Page 49.

Prescrip-tion Book Folio	Cash Received	Details		Medicine	Visits, Consulta-tions,&c.	Amount to Ledger	Folio
	£ s d			£ s d	£ s d	£ s d	
55	..	Allen, Mrs. (Address)	Vis.	..	0 5 0	0 5 0	72
"	1 1 0	Briggs, Miss "	C./d.	..	1 1 0	..	81
"	..	Butt, J. "	Vis.	..	1 1 0	1 1 0	82
"	0 10 6	Spencer, A. "	C./d.	..	0 10 6	..	83
"	..	Jamieson, Miss "	Vis.	..	0 5 0	0 5 0	84
"	0 10 6	Mathias, W. "	Con.	..	0 10 6	..	86

SEPTEMBER 2nd.   Page 50.

Prescrip-tion Book Folio	Cash Received	Details		Medicine	Visits, Consulta-tions,&c.	Amount to Ledger	Folio
55	..	Briggs, Miss (Address)	V. & M.	0 5 0	0 10 6	0 15 6	90
"	0 5 0	Butt, J. "	Do.	0 5 0	1 1 0	1 1 0	91
"	..	Jamieson, Miss "	Vis.	..	0 5 0	0 5 0	98
"	..	Allanson, A. "	Do.	..	0 10 6	0 10 6	99
"	..	Bateson, J. "	Do.	..	1 1 0	1 1 0	100
"	..	North, Mrs. "	Do.	..	0 5 0	0 5 0	101
				£0 10 0	£7 6 0	£7 16 0	

A combined " Prescription and Day Book," and the only form in use which is held to be a combination of " Prescription Book " (giving formulæ, &c.) with a " Summarised Day Book " (for posting purposes), is ruled after the manner of the Summary Book (page 20).

The distinction lies in this fact, that the spaces under each day for each patient are much larger than is necessary in the case of the Summary Book, the intention being that not only cash charges should be entered therein, *but also details of the formulæ of prescriptions* in as terse a form as possible.

This causes the book to be of a very unwieldy size, one month being shown on an opening, and the total for each patient posted monthly to the Ledger. This system is not largely in use, nevertheless it ¦is thought well to mention it in passing.

CHAPTER III.

ANOTHER subject for discussion, whilst dealing with Day Books generally, is as to the best form for recording the details of accounts of "Medical Consultants." In this particular circle of medical men the ordinary Day Book posting system does not apply, as consultants and specialists are, as a rule, remunerated on the spot, and the system of accounts they require is one that merely registers fees, and, of course, also records the professional details of each case. A useful form of book is the following, and, so far as accountants are concerned, it is the only book in this connection that need be discussed.

CONSULTANTS' DAY BOOK.

(Month and Year). Page .

Case No. 37. Date........ .	Particulars of Case	Expenses	Fees	Cash Received
Medical Man...................		£ s d	£ s d	£ s d
Address				
Patient........				
Details......................				
....	Expenses........			
Previous Ref............	....			
Next Ref...............	.... £	....		
Case No. 38. Date..........	Particulars of Case	&c.		

The totals of "Cash Received" can be carried periodically to the consultant's Private Cash Book, and for this purpose the column recording this, as also that for Expenses, are easily added, and can be posted *en bloc*. The difference at any time shown between the "Fees" column and the "Cash" column will give the consultant's outstanding book debts, and these can be taken out and listed at any balancing date. An alternate method is to insert a column for "Date of Cash Received," and utilise the above book as a Cash Book as well as a book of professional record.

Before leaving the subject of Day Book systems, it is now intended to give a specialised system of posting in connection with a "Combined Day Book and Ledger." This is particularly suitable for the recording of "Current Accounts," and in some practices will be found useful as the basis of posting.

The ruling is as follows:—

COMBINED DAY BOOK AND LEDGER FOR CURRENT ACCOUNTS.

Month of...............

Patient's Name	Address	Balance		1	2	3	4	5	6	7	8	&c. to	27	28	29	30	31	£ s d	Month's Fees £ s d	Month's Discount, &c. £ s d	Dates Cash Received	Month's Cash £ s d	Balance £ s d
												VISITS, MEDICINES, &c.											
Abrahams, J...	&c.	£2 2 0	Visits	5/-		5/-	5/-	5/-									5/-	1 0 0	1 4 6		29	0 10 0	2 15 0
			Med.		1/6				1/6	1/6								0 4 6					
			Cash																				
Dyson, A.	&c.		Med.		2/-	2/-	2/-	2/-							2/-	2/-			0 6 0			0 1 6	
			Cash			2/-	2/-																
Ball, R.	&c.	0 10 0	Cash		✳ 1/6	✳ 1/6		✳ 1/6	✳ 1/6					X			✳ 1/6		1 11 0			0 6 0	1 15 0
Dunn, J. B.	&c.		Special					12/-											2 2 0			0 6 0	2 2 0
French, J.	&c.		Con./d.																0 5 0				0 5 0
Totals		£2 12 0																	£5 8 6			£1 3 6	£6 17 0

It will be observed from the above that this Ledger is adaptable to all forms of entry (whether in figures or marks), and also that it is capable of easy proof. For instance, in the above illustration—

The Balances at beginning of Month are .. £2 12 0
Add to this Month's Charges 5 8 6
£8 0 6

And the total equals the Cash received over the Month £1 3 6
Plus the Balances at the end 6 17 0
£8 0 6

As before stated, this Combined book is suitable for current accounts—*i.e.*, particularly accounts which run from month to month. It can, however, be adapted to the ordinary "one-visit" accounts, provided such temporary balances, instead of being carried forward in the Ledger, are transferred each month end to another "Accounts Outstanding" Ledger, which should for convenience of reference be made up on the "Index" system (all accounts of one initial letter being placed together). If this were carried out properly, and a column provided to enable references to such transfers to be made, it is quite possible for the medical man to have all his accounts contained (1) on the Current Accounts Opening, or (2) in the Accounts Outstanding Ledger, as suggested. This certainly enables the quick location of accounts to be accomplished, and it will be appreciated on that account.

FILING SYSTEMS.

(A). "Card Ledger" System (U.S.A.).—

Reference is made to this system in passing, though it will be found in operation to be much too cumbersome, and entailing too much labour, for the great body of English practitioners.

As, however, its essential features, wholly or in part, may be usefully applied to practices requiring a special system (on account of phenomenal number of patients, &c.), such are briefly given.

In a box sufficiently large to contain them, cards, each of which has a tab affixed, are arranged. These cards are duly superscribed, one for each patient, and special cards are also provided for such heads as " Doubtful," " Being recovered," &c. The cards should be slightly less in length than the box containing them, and are usually about $7\frac{1}{2}$ inches by 5 inches.

The distinguishing feature of this system is, primarily, that it claims to provide a means for classifying the patients more definitely and in greater detail than is possible under any other system. Where this necessity for detailed classification is paramount, this system should be considered, as, no doubt, in the United States, such necessity is this system's originating and justifying cause.

The arrangement of the cards can be extended not only into the ordinary alphabetical order, but further into " vowel " subdivisions. " Places " and " suburbs," as also " streets," can also become a part of the basis of classification. When properly arranged, it is claimed that the cards are in themselves a complete index, and also a proper Ledger record. Another advantage claimed is that more than one person can consult the Ledger at once. On the other hand, cards may be lost or become displaced, and the practitioner who entered on this system would almost of necessity require the services of a special clerk to write up and arrange his accounts from day to day.

The ruling of the cards should, of course, allow for columns to record the dates, details, and amounts of charges, and provision would need to be made for cash entries, &c., in accord with his other books of account.

(B). File System.—

This is an English modification of the foregoing, and is very useful in large practices. It is carried out as follows :—

The Visiting List and Prescription Book are entered up in the usual way, but instead of the mass of items being posted directly into the Ledger, the same are carried daily, weekly, or monthly to loose sheets confined in alphabetical order in an ordinary file. Each patient's sheet is filed, of course, under its distinctive initial letter, the file being of the " Index " pattern, and the vowel method of subdivision may also be utilised. At recognised periods, or when the file is full, these Memorandum Accounts are totalled up and the balances transferred to the Ledger. At the same time the file is closed, dated, and a fresh one commenced for a new period. The great advantages of this method are that it saves a great deal of Ledger space, and, moreover, divides the Patients' Accounts up into recognised periodical sections, making reference to specific dates an easy matter.

The following form of ruling for the loose sheets enables the charges in the case of each patient to be analysed into " Visits," " Medicines," &c., though a common plan is to use the ordinary form of Ledger Account.

Name and Address.   Ledger Folio.

Date	Charges					Remarks	Cash Received		
	Con.	Visit	Med.	Sp.	Charges		Date		Amount
					£ s d				£ s d

PART II.

INCOME AND EXPENDITURE.

A medical man's income from professional sources is, of course, derived from patients and public bodies. Owing to the fact, however, of having his professional base at his private establishment, his cash records, private and professional, are very liable to become entangled. Now, it is of prime importance to medical men that their professional cash takings should be kept distinct, as in the event of a sale of practice "Takings" are very generally considered as the basis of the valuation of goodwill. This fact has, then, to be kept in mind in any design for a medical man's Cash Book. A further fact must also be kept in view—viz., the analysis of the medical man's expenditure. No Nominal Ledger Accounts are, of course, necessary, nor yet a Purchase Book, for it will be found that purchases are limited to three or four broad heads of expenditure. To meet these requirements it will be found that a Cash Book with suitable columns for the analysis of the medical man's expenditure, and one also which allows of the private receipts and expenditure being kept separate and distinct from purely professional items, will best meet the case.

The following ruling will be found useful:—

CASH RECEIVED.

Dr.

Date	From whom Received	Leger Folio	Discount Allowed	Items Received	Analysis		
					Patients	Special	Bank

CASH PAID.

Cr.

Date	To whom Paid	Ledger Folio	Discount Received	Items Paid	Analysis			
					Private	House	Coach-man, &c.	Bank

As to the heads of analysis, this can be left to the practitioner's option. Some medical men have "assistants," but not all. With some, expenses of "Horses and Coachman" are heavy; with others comparatively light. All buy drugs, yet with some many purchases are made (small quantities being bought); with others, who buy from one or two firms only, the entries under this head are few. It will be of value, however, in every case to have a column set apart for Capital Expenditure, for in the course of a year a medical man is bound to have certain transactions in Horses, Vehicles, Surgery Fittings, or Instruments, all which should be kept distinct from the ordinary expenses of the practice. "Rent, Rates and Taxes," too, is a head which, being in part chargeable against profits in income tax assessments, should be easily ascertainable when occasion demands.

As to the column headed "Private," it is not at all necessary for *particulars* of all private expenditure to be entered in the Cash Book. For balancing purposes, however, the correct totals under this head should be brought in. The "House Expenses" column will be found useful in enabling the practitioner to arrive at his total hereunder at balancing dates; or, should he have House Expenses which are directly chargeable against professional income (such as servants employed in surgery, &c.), in this column he can locate and summarise the same. Where the practitioner has a branch surgery he can easily arrive at the annual cost of the same by heading one of the columns on the expenditure side of the Cash Book with the necessary particulars.

At the medical man's option a separate book can be kept exclusively for professional cash receipts and expenditure.

In addition to the General Cash Book, it is strongly recommended that a subsidiary book for the recording of cash receipts from patients be kept. Its advantages are obvious:—

(a) The bulk of the medical man's cash receipts will be found in a separate book, under one head, and can be transferred to the General Cash Book periodically in bulk in one amount.

(b) This subsidiary Cash Book can always be at hand in the surgery, and can be entered up at the time cash is paid in. The General Cash Book, not being confined strictly to patients' cash transactions, cannot in every case be so utilised; nor, indeed, can it be left in the hands of third parties in all cases.

(c) This subsidiary Cash Book, being exclusively a patients' Cash Book, minimises the risk of omission to post charges—i.e., all folio column omissions can be easily detected. Moreover, by its aid alone the Patients' Ledger can be proved, no recourse being necessary to the General Cash Book containing outside entries.

(d) This Cash Book also provides a record of the takings of the practice, complete in itself. This, needless to say, might be of great advantage where testimony for the information of an outsider is concerned.

A good ruling is as follows:—

Dr.   PATIENTS' CASH BOOK.   Cr.

Date	Name and Address	Folio in Patients' Ledger	Discount Allowed	Cash Received	Folio G.C.B. or Ledger	Cash Paid or Transferred
			£ s d	£ s d		£ s d

NOTE.—In practices where there are a large number of small cash consultations the daily *total* of these can be entered in the Patients' Cash Book, and posted to a separate "Cash Consultations Account." An alternative method is to provide the Patients' Cash Book with an additional column on the *Dr.* side. As these transactions do not require posting, the total for any period can be arrived at by simple addition of the special column in the Cash Book.

If ruled in this way, waste in Cash Book pages is obviated. When the cash is handed over to the practitioner the above book is credited, and cash reference made to the General Cash Book, or the Ledger folio given as to where the principal is debited with the cash so disposed.

This book can also be utilised, where necessary, as a daily record of Surgery Expenses, such being entered on the credit side, and duplicated (in total or otherwise) periodically in the General Cash Book.

As before stated, the expenditure of a medical man, being easily divided under certain broad heads, precludes the necessity of having a credit system of posting. The plan generally adopted is to take the actual cash expenditure up to any balancing day, and to estimate what has accrued due, by which means the year's expenditure is arrived at, and the analysis obtained from the Cash Book.

For recording the Credit Accounts, however, when necessary, the following book will be found not only useful, but also productive of very little extra labour:—

CREDIT BOOK OR ACCOUNT.

Date	To whom Paid	C. B. Folio	Cash and Discount	Date of Order	No.	From whom Ordered	Total	Drugs, &c.			Horsekeep			Special	
								T. F.	&c.	W. B. &c.	A. K.	A. M. and S.	W. L.		
			£ s d				£ s d	£ s d	£ s d	£ s d	£ s d	£ s d	£ s d	£ s d	£ s d

This book will show at a glance on balancing day the total owing on Credit Purchase Account, and also the state of account between the practitioner and each individual creditor. The columns for analysis can, of course, be extended to suit the case of each practitioner. If, in posting the cash payments, each cash item goes on the same line as the original entry of purchase, it makes the identification of accounts owing at any date very simple.

In cases where the credit book is brought into use, a special column can be added to the Cash Expenditure Analysis, the total of credit purchases (as per the Credit Book) going to swell the other cash purchases, as shown in the Cash Book analysis columns. The purchases of Drugs, Horsekeep, &c., are not extensive enough to warrant a Day Book record being kept, but a properly numbered and counterfoiled Order Book will certainly be found useful, and will enable a check to be placed by the medical man on invoices rendered. If the practitioner adopts such an Order Book, and passes all credit purchases through the same, such a record will be found to be a duplication of the entries in the Credit Book shown above.

Branch Books of Account.—

Many medical men have branches, sometimes left in charge of an assistant, at other times worked personally along with the headquarters' practice. In most cases these branches are in contiguous districts, and the accounts are passed through the headquarters' books. Where this is the case it will always be advisable to set apart special columns in the Cash Book Analysis for the recording of cash relating to those branches, both in regard to receipts from branch patients and branch expenditure (Assistant, Rent, Rates, Caretaker, &c.). This will be easily accomplished.

Where the branch is situated in another town or village, it is, of course, necessary to have a separate Patients' Ledger and Day Book. This, along with a Branch Cash Book, are all the additional books required to record the branch transactions. Such Branch Cash Book would need to record merely the cash receipts from patients and branch expenses, and the *totals* of this subsidiary book only need be brought into the books at headquarters. Where the branch is near the practitioner's house, and in charge of an assistant, a Daily Return made to the practitioner (in the following form) will obviate the necessity of a separate set of books for such branch. The only necessity in this case would be that all outstanding accounts would need to be paid at the headquarters' surgery, as at that establishment only the records of outstanding accounts would be preserved. This difficulty, however, could be surmounted by the branch being kept posted up from month to month of the exact amounts of outstanding accounts.

BRANCH SURGERY DAILY RETURN.

Day,   Month,   Year.

Patients	Nature of Attendance	£ s d	Ledger Folio

BRANCH EXPENSES

£ s d

BRANCH RECEIPTS

£ s d

Cash Receipts (total) .. .. ..

Patients' Accounts .. .. ..

(Details).

Cash in hand.. .. .. £ s d

Receipts as above .. ..

Less Paid as above ..

Cash in hand .. ..

NOTE.—This Return can also be made into a Weekly Return, in which case the weekly total chargeable to each patient will be in accordance with that shown on Visiting List, Form C (page 3).

The best plan is for the above return to be made up into a manifold book, and the detachable portion sent away each day, leaving the carbon copy as a record for the branch assistant's use as required.

It is now proposed to give the summarised results of a medical man's accounts for a prescribed period, and to show the application of the foregoing rulings and methods of accounting to the same. The accounts of our practitioner not having been audited up to the time of our being called in, need first of all to be reduced into order. On going into matters, we are able to verify the following figures :—

Cash in Bank..	..	..	..	£178 12 9
„ „ hand ..	..	..	..	28 3 6
Accounts Owing :—				
Drugs, H. W. & Co. ..	..	..	£5 14 7	
Instruments, C. & G. ..	..	..	3 2 9	
For Gig, A. B. & S. ..	..	..	38 0 0	
For Rent (one quarter)..	..	..	17 10 0	
Horsekeep, C. B. & S...	..	..	9 19 4	
				74 6 8
Patients' Balances ..	..	..	..	425 3 9
Stocks :—				

One Horse (cost £58 in 1898).
  „   „ („ £42 „ 1899).
Brougham (cost £60), written down to £45.
Gig, new (cost £38).
Saddlery and Stable Fittings, £27 19s. 5d.
Stock of Drugs, &c., £30 (approximate).
Stock of Surgery Fittings and Instruments, £147 12s. 6d.

Our first duty, having got these rough figures out, is to deal with them to enable us to get a " starting balance." To this end we deal with the items individually, commencing with :—

Cash in Bank and on hand.—These figures we are able to confirm without trouble.

Horses.—The values given are £58 and £42 = £100. These items need depreciating, which depreciation we accordingly write off at the rate of 10 per cent. per annum, reducing the figures by the sums of £11 12s. od. and £4 4s. od. respectively.

Vehicles.—Brougham : We find this asset has been depreciated, so allow it to stand.

Gig : As this is newly purchased we enter it at cost figure.

Saddlery and Stable Fittings.—We find on investigation that the figures given hereunder are the figures representing the practitioner's expenditure under this head since commencing practice. We therefore write off at the rate of 10 per cent. per annum, and reduce the total to £20 6s. 5d.

Stock of Drugs, Medicine Bottles, &c.—This item of stock is found to keep at a certain level of value, so we take the approximate figure given to us—viz., £30—as representing its capital equivalent. It is not usual to take a detailed stock of this asset, but any substantial fluctuations must be noticed in the accounts, and additions or deductions made as may be necessary.

Surgery Fittings and Instruments.—The figures given hereunder represent the total expenditure under this head. For a commencing figure we deduct depreciation (at 5 per cent.) and reduce the amount to £110, made up as follows : —

Fittings	..	..	..	£75	0	0
Instruments		..	..	35	0	0
				£110	0	0

Outstanding Accounts.—These are Ledger Balances, and are accepted as they stand, after confirmation by the " Invoices rendered."

Patients' Balances.—This amount, £426 3s. 9d., represents the total amount owing as shown by the books. As there is a somewhat large leakage in the medical profession of accounts collectable, it is the accountant's duty to write off from the gross total a reasonable amount for provision against the contingency of loss through bad and doubtful debts. We find the results to come out as follows:—

Good	..	..	..	£341	8	9
Doubtful ..	..	..		46	3	2
Bad	..	..	..	37	11	10
				£425	3	9

We reduce this amount to £347 7s. 11d. by the following allowances:—

50 per cent. on Doubtful Debts	..	..	£23	1	7
100	do.	Bad Debts ..	..	..	37	11	10
5	do.	Good Debts (for Discount)..		17	2	5
			£77	15	10

At the same time the *absolutely* bad debts are written off from the Ledger.

We have now got out all the figures necessary to enable us to construct a Balance Sheet at January 1st 1900. This we now give:—

BALANCE SHEET, 1st January 1900

Liabilities	£	s	d
Capital Account	807	7	11
Accounts owing	74	6	8
	£881	**14**	**7**

Assets	£	s	d	£	s	d
Stocks as follows—						
Drugs	£30	0	0			
Fittings and Instruments ..	110	0	0	140	0	0
Horses, Vehicles, &c.—						
Horses	84	4	0			
Vehicles	83	0	0			
Saddlery	20	6	5	187	10	5
Patients, Accounts owing by ..	387	11	11			
Less Provision.. ..	40	4	0	347	7	11
Cash in Bank				178	12	9
Cash in hand				28	3	6
				£881	**14**	**7**

Under each particular head we now open accounts in the medical man's Private Ledger, and lay down the following system of accounts:—

(*a*) Visiting List (as shown).

(*b*) Day Book, one of the types hereinbefore suggested.

(*c*) Patients' Ledger.

(*d*) Cash Book.

(*e*) Credit Book or Account for Purchases.

At the year-end we are called in make up the practitioner's accounts, and to this end complete the entries for the period, checking them as may be necessary. The following are the summarised books for the year under review:—

DAY BOOK.

Prescription Book Reference	Details (Nature of Professional Work).		Amount Charged	Ledger Folio
	Attendance, &c, .. £ : :			
	Medicine .. .. £ : :		£2,078 3 6	

Dr. CASH

Date	From whom Received	Ledger Folio	Discount Allowed £ s d	Items Received £ s d	Analysis — Bank £ s d	Private £ s d	...Patients £ s d	Special £ s d
	SUMMARY OF ENTRIES FOR YEAR							
1900 Dec. 31	Cash in hand	..	..	28 3 6	178 12 9			
" "	" Bank	..	..					
1901 Dec. 31	Private Receipts	..	55 2 6	125 10 0		125 10 0		
"	Fees from Patients	..		1,685 7 6			1,685 7 6	
"	Special Fees, &c. (Sale of Gig)	..		35 0 0				35 0 0
"	Drawn from Bank	..		1,845 17	1,686 11 6			
"	Paid to do.	..		2 19 0				
"	Cash from Bank (Cash Disbursements)	..						
	Totals ..	..	£52 2 6	£3,722 17 6	£1,865 4 3	£125 10 0	£1,685 7 6	£35 0 0

Cr. BOOK.

Date	To whom Paid	Ledger Folio	Discount Received £ s d	Items Paid £ s d	Analysis — Bank £ s d	Private £ s d	Credit Accounts £ s d	Assistant £ s d	House £ s d	Coachm'n &c. £ s d
	SUMMARY OF ENTRIES FOR YEAR									
	Private Payments over period	..	..	1,579 18 7		1,579 18 7				133 10 4
	Credit Accounts Paid	..	10 12 2	61 4 7			61 4 7			78 3 0
	Cash Expenditure	..		364 0 4				125 0 0	105 10 0	31 8 5
									Coachman	12 6 6
									Travelling	11 12 5
	Paid to Bank	..		1,686 11 6	1,845 17 6				Sundries	
	Received from Bank	..			2 19 0				Repairs ..	
	Do. do. (Cash Disbursed)	..								
1901 Dec. 31	Cash in hand	..		31 2 6	16 7 9					
"	Do. Bank	..								
	Totals ..	..	£10 12 2	£3,722 17 6	£1,865 4 3	£1,579 18 7	£61 4 7	£125 0 0	£105 10 0	£133 10 4

CREDIT BOOK OR ACCOUNT.

All money columns are in £ s d.

Date	To whom Paid	C.B. Folio	Amount Paid and Discount	Date Ordered	Order No.	Amount	Drugs — H. W. & Co.	Drugs — C. & G.	Drugs — R. & S.	Horsek'p — C. B. & Son.	A. B. & S. (Gig)	Special — Rent, &c.	Special — Re-pairs	Special — Fittings
1900 Dec. 31	Balances owing	:	..	..	:	74 6 8	5 14 7	3 2 9	..	9 19 4	38 0 0	17 10 0		
Jan. 3	Rent Paid	:	17 10 0	Goods Ordered over Year	:	217 1 6	28 10 0	..	12 18 6	95 3 0	37 10 0	2 10 0	8 5 0	32 5 0
Feb. 27	A. B. & S.	:	38 0 0			291 8 2	34 4 7	3 2 9	12 18 6	105 2 4	75 10 0	20 0 0	8 5 0	32 5 0
June 21	H. W. & Co.	:	5 14 7											
	Totals	:	61 4 7	Cash Paid	:	61 4 7	5 14 7	..	..	..	38 0 0	17 10 0		
1901 Jan. 1	Balances owing	:	..	..	:	230 3 7	28 10 0	3 2 9	12 18 6	105 2 4	37 10 0	2 10 0	8 5 0	32 5 0

The BANK BOOK shows the following:

1900			£ s d	1900			£ s d
Dec. 31	Cash drawn	..	1,845 17 6	Jan. 1	Cash in Bank	..	178 12 9
"	Do.	..	2 19 0	Dec. 31	Do. to Bank	..	1,686 11 6
"	Cash in Bank	..	16 7 9				
			£1,865 4 3				£1,865 4 3

We note, on going through the books, the following extraordinary items, of which we take due memoranda:—

Capital Items.—

Gig sold for £35 0s. 0d. Another bought for £37 10s. 0d. in November 1900. £35 appears in C. B. " special " column ; £37 10s. in Credit Book.

Surgery fittings increased. Amount of invoice £32 5s. 0d. (not yet paid). This item in Credit Book.

Field rented at £10 per annum. One quarter due. Balance shown in Credit Book.

Stack of hay bought. Most of it consumed. (Item included in Credit Book in amount £95 3s. 0d.)

Drug stocks increased, say, £5 0s. 0d.

The Debtors' Ledger, having been kept on the Summary Book system, is capable of proof, and we therefore summarise it as follows:—

DEBTORS' LEDGER SUMMARY.

			£	s	d					£	s	d
1899 Dec. 31	To Total Balances owing	..	387	11	11	1900 Dec. 31	By Total Fees received..	..	..	1,685	7	6
1900 Dec. 31	" Do. Bills rendered ..	..	2,078	3	6	"	" do. Discount allowed ..	..	..	55	2	6
						"	" do. Balances owing at date	..		725	5	5
			£2,465	15	5					£2,465	15	5

SUSPENSE ACCOUNT FOR DOUBTFUL DEBTS AND DISCOUNTS.

			£	s	d
1899 Dec. 31	By Provision allowed	..	40	4	0

It is now a very easy matter to get out a Trial Balance, as follows : —

TRIAL BALANCE, 31st December 1900.

Reference							£	s	d	£	s	d
Cap. A/c. ..	Capital Account ..	..	..	..	..		647	0	8			
P. & L. A/c.	Discounts Allowed	..	..	..	..		55	2	6			
Stock A/c...	Special Receipts ..	..	..	..			..			35	0	0
P & L. A/c.	Assistant ..	..	..	..	..	..	125	0	0			
Do. ..	House Expenses ..	..	..	..	..		105	10	0			
Do. ..	Travelling Expenses	..	..	..	..		31	8	5			
Do. ..	Cash Purchases ..	..	..	..	..		12	6	6			
Do. ..	Coachman, &c. ..	..	..	..	..		78	3	0			
Do. ..	Repairs ..	..	..	..	..		11	12	5			
Cash A/c...	Balance ..	..	..	..	..		31	2	6			
Bank A/c...	„ ..	..	..	..	..		16	7	9			
Drs. A/c. ..	Total Debtors ..	..	..	..	..		725	5	5			
Cr. Book ..	„ Creditors ..	..	..	..			..			230	3	7
Stock A/c...	Stocks at January 1st 1900		..	..	..		327	10	5			
Cr. Book ..	Credit Purchases—											
P. & L. A/c.	Drugs ..	..	..	£41	8	6						
Do. ..	Horsekeep	..	..	95	3	0						
Stock A/c...	Gig Bought	..	..	37	10	0						
P. & L. A/c.	Rent (Field)	..	..	2	10	0						
Do. ..	Repairs ..	..	..	8	5	0						
Stock A/c...	Fittings ..	..	..	32	5	0						
				217	1	6						
Drs. A/c. ..	Total Bills Rendered	..	..	..	..		..			2,078	3	6
Sus. A/c. ..	Provision for Debts and Discounts		..	..	..		..			40	4	0
							£2,383	11	1	£2,383	11	1

The Stock Account, when written up, shows the following :—

STOCK ACCOUNT.

		Drugs	Fittings	Horses	Vehicles	Saddlery	Total
		£ s d	£ s d	£ s d	£ s d	£ s d	£ s d
1899 Dec. 31	Total Stocks £327 10s. 5d.	30 0 0	110 0 0	84 4 0	3 0 0	20 6 5	327 10 5
1900 Dec. 31	Additions over Year	5 0 0	32 5 0		37 10 0		74 15 0
"	Sales over Year	35 0 0	142 5 0	84 4 0	120 10 0 / 35 0 0	20 6 5	402 5 5 / 35 0 0
"	Depreciation written off		14 4 6	8 8 4	85 10 0 / 8 11 0	2 1 0	367 5 5 / 33 4 10
	Total Stocks at December 31 1900 £334 0 7	35 0 0	128 0 6	75 15 8	76 19 0	18 5 5	334 0 7

Analysis

DEPRECIATION ACCOUNT.

		£ s d			£ s d
1900 Dec. 31	To Amount written off—		1900 Dec. 31	By Increase in Drugs	5 0 0
	Horses	8 8 4		" Balance to Profit and Loss Account	28 4 10
	Gigs, &c.	8 11 0			
	Saddlery	2 1 0			
	Fittings	14 4 6			
		£33 4 10			£33 4 10

PROFIT AND LOSS ACCOUNT.

Dr.   Cr.

	£ s d	£ s d		£ s d
1900 Dec. 31			1900 Dec. 31	
To Purchases—			By Bills Rendered over Year	2,078 3 6
Drugs	41 8 6			
Sundries	12 6 6			
Horsekeep	95 3 0	148 18 0		
„ Expenses—				
House (Rent, &c.) ..	105 10 0			
Rent of Field.. ..	2 10 0			
Assistant	125 0 0			
Coachman, &c. ..	78 3 0			
Repairs (Credit Book)	8 5 0			
Travelling Expenses ..	31 8 5			
Repairs (Cash) ..	11 12 5	360 8 10		
„ Depreciation		28 4 10		
„ Discount allowed ..		55 2 6		
„ Bad Debts written off		88 3 5		
		680 17 7		
„ Net Profit—to Capital Account		1,395 5 11		
		£2,078 3 6		£2,078 3 6

CAPITAL ACCOUNT.

Dr.   Cr.

		£ s d				£ s d
1900				1900		
Dec. 31	To Cash drawn	1,579 18 7		Jan. 1	By Balance at date..	807 7 11
1901				"	" Cash added (private)	125 10 0
Dec. 31	" Balance of Capital	748 5 3		Dec. 31	" Balance from Profit and Loss Account ..	1,395 5 11
		£2,328 3 10				£2,328 3 10
				1901		
				Jan. 1	By Balance of Capital	748 5 3

BALANCE SHEET at December 31st 1900.

Liabilities.

		£ s d
Capital Account		748 5 3
Sundry Creditors		230 3 7
		£978 8 10

Assets.

	£ s d	£ s d
Stocks—		
Drugs	35 0 0	
Fittings	128 0 6	
Horses	75 15 8	
Vehicles	76 19 0	
Saddlery	18 5 5	334 0 7
Sundry Debtors	725 5 5	
Less Provision for Bad and Doubtful Debts	128 7 5	596 18 0
Cash on hand		31 2 9
" in Bank		16 7 9
		£978 8 10

NOTES ON ACCOUNTS.

Bank Account.—

No Bank charges have been brought in, in this instance.

Trial Balance.—

It will be observed that the Trial Balance, being got out in form shown, does away with the necessity for any of the usual Nominal Accounts. In the case of medical men these are hardly necessary. The amount of Capital, £647 0s. 8d., is the balance of Capital Account before the profit for the period is transferred thereto.

Suspense Account.—

On writing off for Bad Debts the sum of £128 7s. 5d., as shown in the Balance Sheet, this Account will be dealt with as follows :—

SUSPENSE ACCOUNT.

Dr.		£	s	d		Cr.	£	s	d
1899 Dec. 31	To Provision for Doubtful Debts and Discounts	128	7	5	1899 Dec. 31	By Balance of Account	40	4	0
					"	" Bad Debts written off	88	3	5
		£128	7	5			£128	7	5
					1901 Jan. 1	By Provision at date	128	7	5

Discount received, £10 12s. 2d. (C.B.). This Discount does not appear in Profit and Loss Account because the *net* Cash Expenditure is treated therein; *i.e.*, £364 0s. 4d., and not £374 12s. 6d.

PART III.

INCOME TAX.

A medical man's professional income is, of course, assessable under Schedule " D." If the total income from all sources does not equal £160 per annum the practitioner is exempt from tax.

From £160 to £400 there is an abatement of £160
 ,, £400 ,, £500 ,, ,, ,, £150
 ,, £500 ,, £600 ,, ,, ,, £120
 ,, £600 ,, £700 ,, ,, ,, £70

Before dealing with aspects of a medical man's income other than professional, we will consider the many points bearing on the computation of the amount of income actually earned by him which is assessable for tax. Perhaps the best method of attaining this object will be to discuss the preparation of accounts from actual figures. For this purpose we append accounts of B. M. Esq., M.B., for the year ended the 31st December 1900, showing for the sake of discussion full details of accounts and analyses of same.

PROFIT AND LOSS ACCOUNT, year ended 31st December 1900.

	£	s	d		£	s	d
HEAD ESTABLISHMENT				Bills Rendered over year ..	1,450	3	6
CHARGES—				Discounts allowed	5	10	2
(1) Rent	65	0	0				
(2) Rates	16	5	0				
(3) Servants	52	0	0				
(4) Repairs	12	0	0				
SURGERY EXPENSES—							
(5) Assistant	120	0	0				
(6) Drugs, &c.	32	0	0				
(7) Fittings altered ..	3	2	6				
HORSEKEEP, &C.—							
(8) Coachman	70	0	0				
(9) Horsekeep	68	0	0				
(10) Repairs (Saddlery)	6	7	2				
MOTOR—							
(11) Motor Repairs ..	12	6	3				
(12) Stationery	4	2	0				
BRANCH SURGERY—							
(13) Caretaker	60	0	0				
(14) Rent	20	0	0				
(15) Rates	5	0	0				
(16) Repairs	3	2	6				
(17) Depreciation, Stocks, &c.	45	0	0				
(18) Bad Debts written off	39	14	6				
(19) Doubtful Debts (estimated loss) ..	14	10	0				
(20) Discounts allowed ..	72	3	2				
Profit	735	0	7				
	£1,455	13	8		£1,455	13	8

INCOME TAX ACCOUNT AS MADE OUT FOR THE COMMISSIONERS.

			£	s	d
Profit for year ended 31st December 1898 ..			435	18	5
,, ,, ,, 1899 ..			600	18	0
,, ,, ,, 1900 ..			710	2	3
Total divided by " 3 "..			3)1,746	18	8

Gives as the average Profit for the last
   three years £582 0 0

which amount is that for which the practitioner is
assessable for tax.

The reduction in the case we have under review is in the sum of £24 1s. 11d., made up as follows :—

		£	s	d
Profit shown by professional Profit and Loss Account		735	0	7
Add—	£ s d			
Item No. 1	21 13 4			
,, ,, 2	5 8 4			
		27	1	8
Deduct—		762	2	3
Item No. 5		52	0	0
Leaving Assessable Amount		£710	2	3

It is now proposed to deal with each item separately, and discuss them each in relation to Income Tax.

Item 1.—House Rent.—

As a medical man's place of residence is also his professional base, he is entitled to charge against his professional income (not more than) two-thirds of his rent. This will be accepted by the bodies of Income Tax Commissioners generally ; though it must be said that, as these gentlemen have absolute option of acceptance, there may be cases in which but one-third of the rent will be allowed to be charged against earnings.

Item 2.—Rates and Taxes.—

This item is the *total* of local rates and taxes. Income tax paid is not allowed to be charged against income for income tax assessment, but is reckoned as a private expense. The proportion of rates and taxes deductible from earnings is reckoned *pari passu* as rent is allowed—viz., generally two-thirds.

Item 3.—Servants.—

The total of Wages hereunder is £156 per annum, and, as of the three, *one* is *exclusively* employed by the medical man on his professional work, the wages of such are charged against gross earnings. The Income Tax Commissioners will generally allow this, in cases where three or four servants are in one employment.

Item 4.—Repairs.—

This is the total of Repairs to Surgery Fittings, &c., and does not, of course, include domestic repairs, which are not chargeable.

Item 5.—Assistant.—

This is, of course, chargeable. The general basis of agreement as to remuneration made between a medical man and his assistant is one usually comprising a question of salary *plus* board and lodging. As this expense is professional *in toto*, £52 has been estimated as the approximate cost of such board and lodging, and charged accordingly. Where the Commissioners object to this arrangement, it can be overcome by the medical man paying his assistant an inclusive salary, and the cash for board and lodging being repaid to the medical man month by month.

Item 6.—Drugs and Bottles.—

This is the total expenditure over the year under this head. When the stock of drugs has increased over the period, the amount charged against Income under the head of Depreciation is reduced. Under the present head, therefore, we charge it in full.

Item 7.—Fittings Altered.—

This is for alterations not necessarily increasing the capital value of the dispensing room, and, being an entirely professional expense, is charged against gross Income. Of course, where the values are increased by these additions, the charge would not in theory be allowable.

Item 8.—Coachman (and Travelling Expenses).—

As a groom or coachman is a necessity to most practitioners the total wages and expenses hereunder are charged against Income. Licences for carriages and male servants are included under "Expenses." As the medical man in the account of earnings has returned the gross amounts of such, it is but just that all expenses of whatever kind connected with his professional "rounds" should be chargeable against Income for assessment purposes.

Item 9.—Horsekeep.—

Hay, Corn, Stable Requisites, Rent of Fields for Horses, &c., are chargeable in full. Where, however, the medical man has a vehicle for exclusively private use, a proportion of such expenses will not be allowed. Where the horses and groom are used for personal as well as professional purposes, the best plan is to take a two-thirds proportion of the total expenses under the heads of "Coachman," "Horsekeep," &c., and reckon one-third as being personal, and consequently not chargeable.

Item 10.—Saddlery Repairs.—

Remarks anent Item 9 apply here also.

Item 11.—Repairs, Motor.—

This should be treated the same as Vehicular Expenses (Item 8).

Item 12.—Stationery.—

This is chargeable, being for professional note-heading, envelopes, &c. *Private* stationery is, of course, not so chargeable.

Item 13.—Caretaker at Branch.—

In this case the sum of £60 covers all the expenses of caretaking at surgery, and is wholly chargeable. against gross Income. If the arrangement had been one based on the caretaker receiving a salary *plus* house expenses, there would be the additional item of " Caretaker's Expenses " likewise chargeable.

Items 14, 15, and 16.—Branch Rent, Rates, and Repairs,

being exclusively professional expenditure, are charged in full against gross Income.

Item 17.—Depreciation.—

" No deductions are allowed for wear and tear of machinery and plant, but allowances may be claimed in respect of those items."

In the " Claim for Allowance " in Assessment Schedule, the value of machinery and plant has to be stated, as also the amount claimed for " wear and tear."

On the other hand, the Commissioners allow for all Repairs and Renewals. The depreciating stocks of the medical man are Horses, Vehicles, Surgical Fittings, Saddlery, and Harness. If reasonable depreciation is disallowed under these heads, the only recourse the medical man has is to take care to charge as much as he legitimately can of his expenditure on practice necessaries (Saddlery, Instruments, Fittings, &c.) against Profit and Loss Account direct, under the head of " Renewals and Repairs." The wear and tear of horses and vehicles is in many cases such as to warrant, not a depreciation of 5 per cent. (which is the claim usually accepted by the Commissioners), but, say, of 15 per cent.

Items 18 and 19.—Bad Debts and provision for Doubtful Debts.—

Before closing his yearly accounts, the medical man will do well to write off all worthless book debts. He will also be wise in transferring all doubtful ones to one account. The Commissioners usually allow him to write off all bad debts against Income, and also to make a reasonable provision for doubtful ones.

Item 20.—Discounts Allowed.—

The practitioner, having credited his Profit and Loss Account with the gross bills due, or sent out, is entitled to write off against Income for assessment purposes the whole of "Discounts allowed" by him to his patients.

Life Insurance Premiums.—

Should the medical man be insured in a British life office, he should make his claim in the orthodox manner by filling up the space provided in the Schedule D Return. The tax on the amount of premium will be deducted from the amount payable on the Demand Note, provided the receipts for such premium have been shown to the Surveyor of Taxes. Otherwise, and if for more than the current year, a form must be obtained from the local Inland Revenue Office, filled up, and forwarded with the premium receipts to the Secretary, Inland Revenue, Somerset House. The claim may be made for three years, and the repayment does not affect the relief granted on incomes under £700. Life insurance premiums are only deductible up to one-sixth of the income assessed.

Besides the assessment of income tax under Schedule D, the following further assessments are made.

Schedule A.—

This is known as *the Landlord's Property Tax*. This is deductible from the rent, and the landlord is bound to allow it under penalty.

Schedule B.—Tenant Farmers' Income Tax.—

Chargeable on one-third the amount of rent. Tenants can claim for over-payments, or elect to be assessed under Schedule D. They rarely adopt the latter course.

Schedule C.—

Assessed on annuities payable out of Government funds.

Schedule E.—

Assessed on salaries and fees of public officials, whether in Government offices, the Army and Navy, Civil Service, County or Municipal Corporations, Public Institutions, or the Church. Expenses incurred in the performance of such duties are deductible.

Wife's Income.—

If the income of the wife is from property or investments, the income must be added to that of the husband, notwithstanding any settlements, and in spite of the provisions of the Married Women's Property Act of 1882. Money earned by the wife, if the joint income is under £500, may be separately assessed, so that each may claim abatement or exemption.

Interest on Borrowed Money or on Mortgages.—

In cases of claim for exemption from tax, such interest is deductible from income before assessment. A special form for " declaration " is printed in the schedule. In other cases no deductions are allowed under either of these heads, the duty on such interest or mortgage being deductible from the person to whom the payment is made.

Interest on Capital.—

No allowances are made hereunder.

Partner's Assessment.—

A partner in a practice may be separately assessed for the purpose of claiming abatement or exemption, and a form is provided for this purpose in the return.

Assessment of a new Practice.—

Anyone succeeding to a practice cannot treat it as a new business. The assessment will be continued, unless proof can be given of a falling off of profit from some specific cause. If a practice is commenced within the year of assessment, the profits are to be estimated according to the best of the practitioner's knowledge and belief, and the grounds on which the estimate is based must be stated.

Appeals

re overpayment of tax must be prepared for three years, and the average profit shown. The three years must be the *last* three years up to the 5th of April of the year of assessment— *i.e.*, assessment calculation in our example is on the three years ending December 31st 1898, 1899, and 1890 respectively. The tax is payable for 1901-2. Notice of appeal must be given if the assessment is based on a larger figure than has been returned. If the Surveyor of Taxes is seen, and copies of the Profit and Loss Accounts for the three years are produced, the loss of time involved in an appeal is sometimes obviated. If the appeal is disallowed, there is no higher Court to appeal to against the Commissioners.

Notes on the Collection of a Medical Man's Outstanding Accounts.—

The policy of the old-established practitioner under this head was to be usually very slow in the rendering of accounts to his patients. Quarterly, and even annual accounts were once the rule rather than the exception. Under such circumstances—and even nowadays in certain cases—the practice was to post up the Ledger only at long intervals of time. Times and methods, however, are fast changing, especially in the " general practices " of the cities. Hence these remarks as to methods of collection.

An increasingly popular method among medical men nowadays is to place the collection of a section of their accounts outstanding in the hands of an outsider. In crowded districts, where the practitioner is called in by all types of people, this procedure is especially necessary. Apart from the prevention of bad debts thus brought about, it is acceptable to the busy practitioner, because it saves him much prosaic clerical work, and obviates the necessity of a periodical scrutiny of his Ledger Accounts. The following methods have been practised in this connection, and found of advantage :—

(a) At each month-end the collector receives a list of all accounts which have become due during the month for casual professional services—i.e., " single visit " patients, as opposed to the *regular* ones. These he collects straightway, and, if necessary, is able to place pressure on the several debtors without evil results.

(b) At each quarter-end, accounts, long overdue (say six or twelve months, at the practitioner's discretion), are listed, and it is quite reasonable for the medical man, in view of his quarterly, half-yearly, or annual balancing to have a circular sent out, reminding his debtors of the fact, and appointing a day for the collector to call.

The accounts of his regular patients are, of course, allowed to stand in his Ledger indefinitely, the medical man in such cases receiving from time to time sums on account of each patient's indebtedness.

The commission usually payable for collection varies, of course, according to the difficulties or otherwise surrounding the work. Probably a fair average rate is 5 per cent. inclusive, taking good and bad debts together.

Notes on the Assessment of Practice Values.—

This task comes well within the scope of work of the qualified accountant, and, indeed, none is better qualified to deal with it than he. Possibly the first matter of moment in discussing this question is that of the

BASIS OF ASSESSMENT (OR CAPITALISATION).

The Practice Value is made up of three items. The first is that asset which goes under the name of *Goodwill*. There is no universally accepted rule upon which to found the assessment of the value of goodwill. A very commonly accepted basis is to get out the cash takings for the past three years, and to reckon goodwill as being equal to one year's average of the same. Many practices change hands, however, on a basis of mutual agreement between the vendor and purchaser. The second asset for assessment is that which goes under the heading of *Stocks*. This figure is arrived at on the basis of mutual agreement, or, failing this, is taken at a valuation. The third head—and in arriving at this the accountant is indispensable—is the total amount of outstanding *Book Debts*. In this connection, however, it must be said that the taking over of the balances owing on current accounts is going out of favour, the increasing custom becoming for the outgoing practitioner to retain these, collecting them at his own will and discretion—in most cases probably handing the matter over to his accountant to deal with.

The procedure in assessing the value of goodwill (the *basis* thereof having been mutually agreed to) follows on the following broad lines. Most practitioners, knowing the value of such records in the disposal of a practice, keep a fairly accurate record of their cash receipts. It will fall to the accountant to check these for the three years with which he is concerned. Special care will need to be taken in getting out the memoranda recording allowances: where these are large, the takings may be materially reduced. Bad debts also will need to be taken into view, as also the charges for collection. What the accountant requires is the *net* total of receipts.

An important matter in connection with the assessment of this branch of the Practice Value is to deal correctly with emoluments and official salaries in getting out the average cash takings. Where there is a mutual agreement between the two parties that such salaries and emoluments are to be reckoned in the figures on which the goodwill estimate is based, it is, of course, included. In all other cases (unless the transfer of practice carries with it the undoubted right of succession to such official appointments, and it is mutually agreed upon) such special fees and salaries are not included by the accountant in his Cash Summary for the three years.

As to Stocks of Drugs, Horses, Vehicles, &c., in the absence of mutual agreement, this assessment is a matter more for the licensed valuer than the qualified accountant. What the accountant could do with advantage in relation to Stock is to prepare a Return of the Purchases and Dates in relation to such stock, and, on submitting this to the proposed purchaser, a mutual agreement might be arrived at without recourse to the licensed valuer.

Where it falls to the lot of the accountant to prepare the figures relating to the total of outstanding Book Debts on behalf of the purchasing practitioner, the work is comparatively straightforward. The first necessity is to decide on the exact date of transfer, and to assure oneself that all Day Book and Cash Book entries up to that date are made in the Ledger. Where the Summary Book is used in the scheme of accounts, a proof of the Ledger will, of course, be arrived at.

Having verified the postings from the Visiting List, Prescription Day Book, and Cash Book to the Ledger, it remains for the accountant to extract and tabulate the full list.

The following form of schedule will be found useful in this connection :—

Ledger Folio	Name and Address of Debtor	Amount of Debt	Analysis			Remarks
			Good	Bad	Doubtful	
		£ s d				

NOTES ON BAD AND DOUBTFUL DEBTS.

The Ledgers of most medical men disclose debts which, on account of age, may be considered worthless, being covered by the Statute of Limitations. Others standing in the books bear *primâ facie* evidence of worthlessness, or at any rate inspire doubt as to their value by reason of having been put into collectors' hands, or the debtor having " gone away " or repudiated payment.

For making sure his conclusions, and at the same time utilising a unique opportunity for the collection of outstandings, a very good plan for the accountant to adopt, after scheduling the total debtors, is to circularise each patient, and ask for confirmation or otherwise of the amount recorded. It will be found that this plan will bring in a large proportion of the amount due. Where the exigencies of the situation do not admit of this course, the assessor perforce must rely upon his own discretion and professional skill for arriving at a fair and reasonable assessment. Having written off the wholly bad and provided for the doubtful debts, he will, of course, further discount the sum remaining by a percentage to cover cost of collection and inevitable allowances.

Having arrived at the assessed value of debts outstanding, the stocks also having been valued, and the goodwill arranged satisfactorily, the legal transfer can then be arranged.

ABSTRACT OF THE LAW BEARING ON THE ACCOUNTS OF MEDICAL MEN.

To enable a practioner to recover his fees in a Court of Law he must be "registered." In other senses registration is not compulsory. Unregistered medical men (who must, of course, be "qualified") are fully entitled under the law to open a surgery and to do a "cash" business.

A practitioner with a surgical qualification only cannot recover fees from a patient for attendance in such cases as fever, &c.

A firm of medical men, one partner of which is registered as a surgeon and apothecary, and his partner as a surgeon only, are allowed to recover through the Courts on a joint claim for attendance and medicines supplied in both capacities, even though one member of the firm be unregistered.

Medical men must prove registration in the event of their wishing to prove their claims on a testator's estate, or to sue on a promissory note.

The production of The Medical Register is accepted as *primâ facie* proof of registration, provided such Register contains the necessary entry.

A medical man who has exercised supervision over an unqualified assistant, is entitled to sue for services rendered by such assistant.

An infant may contract with, and so become liable to, a medical man for attendance and medicines.

A wife may pledge her husband's credit for attendance and medicine.

Practitioners' claims in law cannot be disputed on the ground of failure to effect a cure; but the patients have, in come cases, a right of action for negligence.

Medical men's charges, if enforced through the law, must, in the opinion of the Court, be "reasonable."

A bankrupt practitioner may recover for professional attendance and advice.

General Information.—

The medical profession was consolidated and placed upon its modern basis by the "Medical Act" of 2nd August 1858, which Act brought into being the General Council of Medical Education and Registration of the United Kingdom. Amongst the clauses of that Act are the following :—

As to regulation and qualification of practitioners in medicine and
      surgery.
,, the Register and those entitled to registration.
,, examinations and those entitled to sit at same.
,, qualifying bodies.
,, the term "legally qualified practitioner," and those entitled to
      use it.
,, the exemption of medical men from juries and service in the
      militia.
,, appointments open to registered practitioners.
,. the validity of certificates.
,, penalties for false description.
,, rendering accounts to Parliament.

Some dozen minor Acts have been passed since the above, each modify-
ing or extending, in some degree, the provisions of the Act of 1858.

The General Council of Medical Education and Registration of the United Kingdom.—

This Council is constituted by law for the general supervision and
government of the medical profession. At 1st January 1902 the govern-
ing body consisted of President, Sir William Turner, K.C.B., M.B., with
thirty-one additional members representative of the various examining
bodies, the Crown, &c., one General Registrar, three Branch Registrars,
and two Treasurers.

Official Register, entitled "The Medical Register" (published for
the General Council in January of each year by Spottiswoode & Co., 54
Gracechurch Street, E.C.), contains last Registration Returns, text of the
Medical Acts, constitution of the General Council, and a Directory of all
registered qualified medical practitioners, with nature of qualification,
dates relating thereto, &c. Price 6s.; for past years, 2s.

The Medical Directory (published by J. & A. Churchill, 7 Great
Marlborough Street, London) gives an abstract of the law bearing on the
profession, as also a list of practitioners, subdivided into lists for London,
Provincial, Wales, Scotland, and Ireland. Also lists for the Colonies and
foreign registered practitioners. Each medical man's full name, time of
qualifying, nature of qualification, and official appointments given. Price
14s.

Registration Figures at 1st January 1902.

(Per Medical Register)

			Totals from beginning of Registration in 1858 to Jan. 1st 1902			Total in Register at 1st Jan. 1902	
			No.	%		No.	%
England	..	..	39,215	61·72	..	21,022	56·95
Scotland	..	..	14,686	23·11	..	10,803	29·27
Ireland	..	..	9,637	15·17	..	5,087	13·78
Totals ..		..	63,538	100	..	36,912	100

A List of the Qualifications of Medical Men.

Degrees or Abbreviated Qualifications.

A List of the Qualifications of Medical Men.	Degrees or Abbreviated Qualifications.
Royal College of Physicians, London.	Fellow. Member. Licentiate. (R.C.P. Lond.).
Royal College of Surgeons, London.	Fellow. Member. Licentiate (Mid.). (R.C.S. Lond.).
Royal College of Physicians, Edinburgh.	Fellow. Member. Licentiate. (R.C.P. Edin.).
Royal College of Surgeons, Edinburgh.	Fellow. Member. Licentiate. (R.C.S. Edin.).
Faculty of Physicians and Surgeons of Glasgow.	Fellow. Licentiate. (Fac. P. & S. Glas.).
Royal College of Physicians of Ireland.	Fellow. Member. Licentiate. Lic. (Mid.). (R.C.P. Ireland).
Royal College of Surgeons of Ireland.	Fellow. Licentiate. Lic. (Mid.). (R.C.S. Ireland).
Apothecaries Hall of Dublin.	Lic. A H. Dublin.
Do. Society of London.	Lic. S.A. London.
Do. Hall, Dublin.	Lic. A.H. Dublin.
University of Oxford.	M.D. M.B. Lic. Med. Bach. Surg. (Univ. of Oxford).
Do. Cambridge.	M.D. M.B. Lic. Med. Bach. Surg. (Univ. of Cambridge).
Do. Durham.	M.D. M.B. Bach. Surg. Lic. Med. M.S. (Univ. of Durham),
Do. London.	M.D. M.B. Bach. Surg. M.S. (Univ. of London).

Victoria University.		M.D. M.B. Mas. Surg. Bach. Surg. (Victoria Univ.).
University of Birmingham.		M.D. M.B. Bach. Surg. (Univ. of Birmingham).
Do.	Edinburgh.	M.D. M.B. Mas. Surg. Bach. Surg. (Univ. of Edin.).
Do.	Aberdeen.	M.D. M.B. Bach. Surg. Mas. Surg. (Univ. of Aberdeen).
Do.	Glasgow.	M.D. M.B. Bach. Surg. Mas. Surg. (Univ. of Glasgow).
Do.	St. Andrews.	M.D. M.B. Bach. Surg. Mas. Surg. (Univ. St. Andrews).
Do.	Dublin.	M.D. M.B. Lic. Med. Mas. Surg. Bach. Surg. Lic. Surg. M.A.O. (Univ. of Dublin.)
Royal University of Ireland.		M.D. M.B. Mas. Surg. Bach. Surg. M.A.O. (Univ. of Ireland).

INDEX.

80   INDEX.

INDEX OF RULINGS AND PRO FORMA ACCOUNTS.

ADVERTISEMENTS

OF SOME OF THE

MORE IMPORTANT WORKS

PUBLISHED BY GEE & CO.

The Accountant.

The Recognised Weekly Organ of Chartered Accountants

AND

Accountancy throughout the World.

The New Volume commences in January.

THE ACCOUNTANT is published weekly, in time for Friday evening's mail, and is the medium of communication between the members of the Institute of Chartered Accountants in England and Wales and Accountants generally throughout the World.

Contents :

Subscriptions :

Yearly .. 24/-	Half-Yearly .. 13/-	Post free, United Kingdom.	
„ .. 26/-	„ .. 14/-	„ Abroad.	

Payable in Advanc

The Accountant.

The Recognised Weekly Organ of Chartered Accountants

AND

Accountancy throughout the World.

Volumes.

To reduce the number of Volumes required for Stock purposes a few of these Volumes will be sold at reduced prices as follows :

1890	..	14/- net	1896	..	14/- net
1891	..	14/- ,,	1897	..	15/- ,,
1892	..	14/- ,,	1898	..	15/- ,,
1893	..	14/- ,,	1899	..	20/- ,,
1894	..	14/- ,,	1900	..	24/- ,,
1895	..	14/- ,,	1901	..	26/- ,,
		1902	..	26/- net.	

CARRIAGE FORWARD.

Order Form.

Date..

To Messrs. GEE & CO.,
    34 Moorgate Street, London, E.C.

Please supply........cop........ of Vol............................

Enclosed is remittance for..........................

Name...

Address...

....

52 PAGES. PRICE 2/6 NET.

𝕳and=𝕭ook to 𝕾tamp

𝕯uties and 𝕽eceipts

BY

H. LAKIN=SMITH, F.C.A., F.S.S.

THIS work has been prepared to meet the requirements of Chartered Accountants, Secretaries of · Limited Companies, House and Estate Agents, and many others by whom a handbook on this important subject has long been needed.

Contains a full Discourse upon Receipts, particulars of Duties and Fees payable on the Registration of Companies. Particulars of the Death Duties, and the Rates and Particulars of all the more important Stamp Duties now in force.

AUDIT NOTE-BOOK

Nos. 1 and 2.

Price 6d. each, or 5s. per dozen.

THE object of these books (which have been compiled in consequence of a suggestion put forward by Mr. (now Lord) Justice Vaughan Williams), is to afford a permanent record of the work actually done in connection with any particular Audit, and of the Queries raised and Answers received thereto, so that the principal may not only know at any time what work was actually performed, but also which members of his staff are responsible therefor.

The NOTE-BOOK is framed to meet the normal requirements of all ordinary industrial undertakings, but is so designed that it may be readily modified to meet the

SPECIAL REQUIREMENTS OF ANY PARTICULAR BUSINESS.

It is suggested that, at the commencement of a new Audit, the principal should himself settle the precise amount of work to be done.

No. 1 AUDIT NOTE-BOOK (for Continuous Audits) provides space for the work done during each month of a year.

No. 2 AUDIT NOTE-BOOK is available for Four Completed Audits, whether Quarterly, Half-yearly, or Annually.

The facts that

OVER 3,000 COPIES HAVE ALREADY BEEN SOLD,

and that among the purchasers are to be numbered many of the **LEADING FIRMS OF CHARTERED ACCOUNTANTS**, are sufficient evidence of the practical character of the AUDIT NOTE-BOOK and of its utility.

The Price per 100 is 40s.,

and purchasers of this quantity are entitled to have their names printed upon the front page free of charge.

NEW EDITION.

100 Pages, Foolscap 4to. Price 2/- per copy, 20/- per doz., or 70/- for 50 copies, £5 10s. for 100 copies.
N.B.—If 50 Copies are ordered, Accountant's Name and Address will be printed on cover.

AUDIT NOTE-BOOK

No. 3.

(FOR IMPORTANT AUDITS.)

In response to the numerous requests which we have received for a larger and more complete AUDIT NOTE-BOOK, so designed as to meet the requirements of Audits relating to **undertakings of any description**, or of a **complicated nature**, we have decided to issue a Third Series of the "AUDIT NOTE-BOOK," which has already been found of such **great utility to the Profession generally.**

This series is so designed as to be suitable for any business—**Manufacturing, Trading, or Financial**—and to undertakings of practically any magnitude, while ample space is also afforded for notes in connection with Audits that are not quite straightforward.

An important feature of the present series is the space provided for entries of Ledger Balances, Trial Balance, &c., rendering the preservation of **loose sheets** (which so easily get mislaid) quite **unnecessary.**

It may be added that Series I. and II. of the "AUDIT NOTE-BOOK," which for some years past hav been regularly used by many of the **leading Firms in the Profession**, and which have been foun most useful for ordinary Commercial Audits (especially when conducted continuously) will continue to b issued as heretofore at the rate of **6d.** per copy, **5s.** per dozen, or **40s.** per hundred.

Orders (accompanied by a remittance) should be forwarded at once to
GEE & Co., Printers & Publishers, Moorgate St., London, E.C.

152 Pages. Demy 8vo.

BOOKKEEPING FOR COMPANY SECRETARIES

Second Edition.	BY LAWRENCE R. DICKSEE, F.C.A.	Price 3/6 net.

THIS Work (which is founded upon a course of lectures delivered under the auspices of the Council of the Institute of Secretaries) deals very fully with those questions in relation to Bookkeeping, a knowledge of which is essential upon the part of every Company Secretary. It will, therefore, be found of the greatest value to all who occupy—or expect to occupy—that position, and also to all Accountant Students.

Price 2s. 6d.

The Cost Accounts OF AN ENGINEER AND IRONFOUNDER.

A REPRINT OF TWO LECTURES READ BEFORE THE SHEFFIELD CHARTERED ACCOUNTANTS STUDENTS' SOCIETY, BY

J. W. BEST, F.C.A.

THE first portion deals with the Engineering and the second with the Foundry Department, and numerous forms of books and accounts are given and explained. The systems advocated are adaptable to both small and large businesses, and show how detailed or aggregate costs and monthly trading results are arrived at and shown.

GEE & CO., Publishers, 34 Moorgate St., London, E.C.

Accountancy and Law Publications.

				Pub. Price NET
Accountant, The.	Weekly			-/6
,,	,,	per annum, post free (U.K.) ...		24/-
		do. do. Foreign ...		26/-
,,	,,	Binding Cases		2/4
,,	,,	File Cases		3/4
Accountants' Journal.	Monthly			-/9
,,	,,	Per annum		7/6
,,	**and Bookkeeper's Vade-Mecum.**	(Whatley)		7/6
,,	**Assistant.** (Beckett) ...	... ...		6/-
,,	**Code** ...	... ...	doz.	5/-
,,	**Compendium.** (Dawson)	... ...		15/-
,,	**Diary.** I.	(Foolscap 1 day to page) ...		8/-
,,	,, II.	(,, 2 ,,) ...		3/6
,,	,, III.	(,, 3 ,,) ...		1/6
,,	,, III.A.	(,, 3 ,,) ...		2/-
,,	,, IV. & IV.F.	(8vo. 1 ,,) ..		5/-
,,	,, V.	(,, 2 ,,) ...		2/6
,,	**Manual.** Vols. I. to VIII.,	...	each	12/6
,,	,, except Vol. III.	...		10/6
,,	,, The set of 8 Vols. ...	...		80/-
Agricultural Accounts. (Meats)	... ...			5/-
Ante-Audit.	... ...	...	each	1/-
,,	... ...	...	½-doz,	5/6
,,	... ...	...	doz.	10/-
Auctioneers' Accounts. (Dicksee)	... ...			3/6
Audit Note Books I. & II.	... ...		each	-/6
,,	,, ,, ...		doz.	5/-
,,	,, ,, ...		100	40/-
,,	,, III.		each	2/-
,,	,, ,, ...		doz.	20/-
,,	,, ,, ...		50	70/-
,,	,, ,, ...		100	110/-

GEE & CO., 34 MOORGATE ST., LONDON, E.C.

	Pub. Price NET
Auditing. (Dicksee) (5th Edition)	21/-
Australian Mining Companies' Accounts. (Godden & Robertson)	3/6
Bank Bookkeeping and Accounts. (Meelboom)	5/-
Bankruptcy. (Stevens) (2nd Edition)	7/6
,, Time Table.	-/6
,, Trustee's Estate Book. (Dicksee)	4/-
,, do. do. doz.	40/-
,, Trustees, Liquidators, and Receivers, Law of. (Willson)	5/-
Bookkeeping, Antiquity of. (Heaps)	1/-
,, Elementary. (Day)	1/-
,, Elements of. (Streeter)	1/6
,, Exercises. (Dicksee)	3/6
,, for Accountant Students. (Dicksee)	10/6
,, ,, Company Secretaries. (Dicksee)	3/6
,, ,, Publishers. (Allen) ...	2/6
,, ,, Retail Traders. (Findlay)	3/-
,, ,, ,, Record Book (Findlay)	4/-
,, ,, Solicitors. (Hodsoll)	3/6
,, ,, Tanning Trade. (Sawyer) ...	2/6
,, ,, Technical Classes and Schools. (Clarke)	2/6
,, ,, Terminating Building Societies. (Lees)	3/6
,, ,, Principles of. (Carlill)	3/6
Builders' Accounts. (Walbank)	3/6
Chartered Accountants' Charges. (Pixley) (2nd Edition)	10/6
Companies Act, 1900. (Reid)	1/-
,, ,, ,, Duties of Auditors under	1/-
Company Secretary. (Fox) (3rd Edition)	20/-
,, Winding-up Time Table	-/6